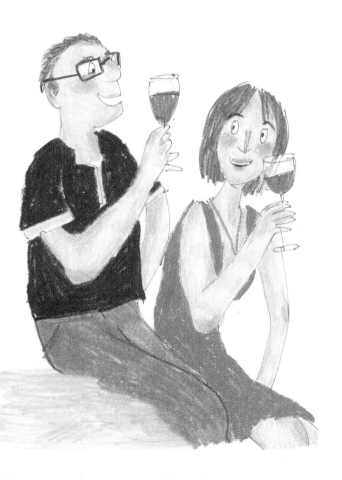

Published by Little Lolly Books 2021
Copyright © Laurence Lee 2021
The moral right of the author has been asserted
ISBN No. 9798455137167
Typeset in Caslon by Bus Stop Editorial Services
Illustrations by Harley Morrison
Edited by Gary Bainbridge

DIABETES
EASY as PIE

Laurence Lee

LITTLE
LOLLY
BOOKS

Foreword

I first met Laurence Lee at Keele motorway service station on the M6, when we were returning from an Everton game in the 1994/95 season.

We had two things immediately in common: we were both Evertonians and we were both disappointed!

As Everton manager at the time, you could say that I was doubly disappointed, but little did I know that this chance meeting was the start of a friendship that still lasts to this day.

Several years later, through Laurence, I was asked to join the Everton Former Players Foundation as a Trustee, a position that I gladly accepted, and still retain.

Our friendship grew and I had the pleasure of dining out with Laurence and his beautiful wife Nichola.

After a great night, and a terrific meal, I never would have guessed that Laurence was diabetic, a revelation that only came to light when I read this book! This book is surely a fantastic example to any unfortunate young person who contracts diabetes, and wants to live a normal life, to never give up.

Laurence went on to take up one of the most fastidious of professions and became a very successful lawyer, most famously as defence solicitor in the James Bulger case.

We never got to enjoy a second meal, as lovely Nichola fell victim to a horrible and debilitating disease only months ago.

I'm sure that Laurence will care for three lovely young ladies — Ella, Frankie, and Natasha — the way that Nichola would have wanted, and continue to be an inspiration to any diabetic, young or elderly.

We still have two things in common, Laurence, my friend: Everton and a smile.

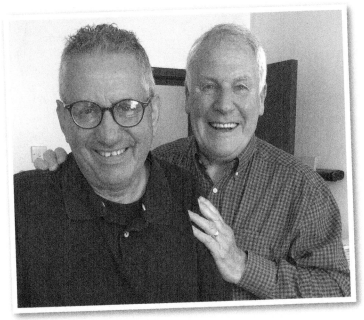

Joe Royle
(Number 9)
July 2021

This book is a perfect example of the sheer volume and variety that can be packed into one lifetime. . . a life lived against the constant presence of Type 1 diabetes and the self-discipline that imposes.

But my friend Laurence vowed when diabetes was diagnosed during his early teens that it would be no obstacle to him and his engaging and humorous story offers irrefutable proof that it has been no such thing, perhaps even a driving force.

His book takes us through the many twists and turns of Laurence's life and career, the light and the dark including his life-long adulation of Everton Football Club — a path that led to him becoming an inspirational chairman of the club's Former Players' Foundation – and a legal career as a highly respected solicitor.

In that role he writes compellingly about his involvement in one of the most chilling child murders of the 20th century, which led to him presenting a revealing television documentary about the custodial differences in the treatment of child offenders between Britain and Scandinavia.

In stark contrast, his legal duties also earned him a place in the Mail on Sunday's Quotes of the Week when, defending a serial streaker, he told the magistrates that "my client has turned over a new fig leaf."

Laurence's ability as a public speaker is reflected in the book's humour and my wife Pat, who served nine years as a Southport councillor, still talks about Laurence's speech at a political fund-raising dinner. "He was so funny the diners didn't want him to stop and didn't want to go home. They were crying with laughter over their dinner plates," she recalls.

The publication of this book follows the untimely and tragic death of Laurence's lovely wife, Nichola. But the lady herself would be proud of how Laurence and their three daughters, Ella, Francesca and Natasha, have responded to the tragedy and fulfilled the adage that life must go on.

And that is certainly NOT easy as pie.

John Keith
Author and broadcaster
July 2021

Introduction

"Positive vibes" has always been my mantra. As the *Monty Python* team sang, always look on the bright side of life. Some might argue that this logic is easier said than done. These are not just idle words, but, having been diagnosed as a Type 1 diabetic at the tender age of 14, an outlook of doom and gloom on my part might have been justified. But I decided that, to quote *The Shawshank Redemption,* my favourite film of all time, I had to make a simple decision: get busy living or get busy dying.

The fact that I'm still here and reasonably fighting fit some 50 plus years later tells you which option I chose.

The aim of this book is to assure fellow Type 1 diabetics that, with the right positive frame of mind, there is nothing to prevent you from leading a full, active, and, above all, a totally normal way of life. In order to achieve this you must first overcome the initial shock of being diagnosed as a diabetic. And then you must create a positive mindset and a determination to overcome everything that this nuisance of a disease may throw at you. That is exactly what diabetes is… a mere nuisance, but only if you control it and don't let it dominate your life

This is the story of how I have achieved this for more than 50 years, albeit with the help, love and guidance of so many individuals in the form of family, friends, and, of course, my medical teams, funded mainly by our brilliant, but overly and unduly criticised NHS.

Laurence Lee
July 2021

1
There Are Places I'll Remember

On 16 January 1968, my life was turned upside down. This was when Dr Heinz Fuld confirmed my worst fears in his surgery at 69 Rodney Street, Liverpool. Having observed my symptoms, he telephoned Sefton General Hospital and uttered words that felt like a dagger through the heart...

Dr Fuld, who was to become my life-long hero, was a refugee from Nazi Germany. My grandfather, too, was a refugee from anti-semitism, but in his case from Russia. Isaac Pikelnovich was in the Russian Army. His party piece was throwing cannonballs. That level of strength and athleticism seems to have been diluted through the genes and generations. These days, I can just about throw a party. But Isaac and his mate, Levi, wanted to escape and head west, hoping to make it to America, the land of opportunity. But they only made it as far as Hull, thinking it was America, like Christopher Columbus actually reaching America and thinking it was India.

Unfortunately, my grandpa's friend, Levi, started getting ill. This, of course, was a time before the National Health Service, before the medical advances of the 20th century that have saved so many lives, including my own. And he was dying. And he told my grandfather his dying wish. He begged him, "Would you take the name Levi and carry it on?"

What would you do? I mean, if you had a name like Pikelnovich, on one level you'd be only too pleased to change it. But this was a

11

chance for a fresh start for my grandad. After all, he'd left his old life behind. So he took the name Levi, in honour of his comrade, and, eventually, he had children, including my father.

My dad, David Levi, was born in Huddersfield in 1915. He was determined to become a doctor, and, in order to achieve that ambition, to attend the University of Leeds. But anti-semitism was rife in those days, particularly in Leeds, and of course he knew he wouldn't get in, so he changed his name to David Lee in 1941. So, with me, there were three generations of men, with three different names. I'm sticking with Lee, by the way. The only time I ever thought of changing it back was when Everton had the manager Gordon Lee in the late 70s. I used to go to the match, and, when he was beginning to fail badly, they were all shouting "Lee out! Lee out!" And my dad put his hand on my shoulder and said, "Don't worry, son, they don't mean us."

But I'm getting ahead of myself. My dad did, in fact, qualify after attending the University of Leeds, and then he lived in Leeds following a distinguished stint in the army during World War II, where he was appointed Captain. He served on troop ships, where his main task was immunising thousands of troops against various diseases. That might explain why he excelled at darts, both in the army and in later life…

Apart from the two occasions when his ship was torpedoed, he didn't have to endure the suffering that so many of his comrades had to go through, thanks to excellent cuisine on board, and his ability to make friends worldwide. His fine injecting technique would help me get used to the many years of self-jabbing that lay ahead of me.

After he was demobbed he commenced his civilian medical career in Leeds. He and his best friend had heard there was a party in Liverpool one Saturday night just after the end of the war. Thank heavens they made it to Liverpool, because it was there he met my dear mum, Hazel Green.

I was born in Oxford Street Maternity Hospital on 2 April 1953, completing David and Hazel Lee's family. My brother Michael had been born four years earlier, and I worshipped him. In many ways, I still do. Incidentally, my oldest friend, Barry Kinshuck, was born at Oxford Street seven days before me. He's a dentist now. I always feel happy when it comes to his birthday because he's a year older than me for a week.

I went to Heatherlea School on Lyndhurst Road, where many Jewish kids went. The headmaster was Major Cole, and it was owned by the Major, along with Mrs Cole. I had happy days at Heatherlea, and when I was six I went to Liverpool College in David House.

That year we moved house. I first lived over my father's surgery on the corner of Storrsdale Road and Mather Avenue. It's still there, but in those days it was so different. You'd go in to see my dad and he'd be smoking. And he was overweight. And a certain patient would come in and he'd say, "You smoke, stop it! And you're overweight, cut out your food!" And he'd be eating chocolate.

We then lived opposite Allerton Manor golf course. This meant that our local synagogue was Allerton. But my grandfather, Sidney Green, was a founder of Greenbank Drive Synagogue, so we went there. I'd walk round there on a Saturday morning, while he'd hypo-critically drive to the synagogue, park half a mile away, and pretend he'd walked.

My maternal grandmother, Edith, like my paternal grandmother, came from Russia. And her English was very broken. She was very religious and I had to go to the synagogue on Saturday, the Sabbath, to keep her happy. I remember once turning up at Greenbank Drive Synagogue wearing a brown suit. I was only about 10 or 11, and my grandfather said, "Excuse me, what are you wearing?"

I said, "I'm wearing a suit."

He said, "It's a brown suit! This is Greenbank Drive Synagogue, not Aintree Racecourse!"

The synagogue was absolutely packed out in those days. On the Day of Atonement - Yom Kippur - they had to have extra seating, because it was so full, and there would be my grandmother, up in the gods, because it was still segregated: women upstairs, men downstairs. And if ever I were caught chatting to the pal next to me, because I didn't want to pay any attention to proceedings, I just wanted to talk about football… well, if looks could kill… the daggers she'd give me, and she'd tap the prayer book, as if to say, "Hey, you, get your head down into that book." And she'd be there from 9.30 in the morning until the fast ended at eight o'clock at night. You know, I'd roll up at 11am, bugger off for lunch at 1pm, and she wouldn't move, so she thought I was a complete and utter heathen. And she was right.

It's heartbreaking to see the state of that synagogue now. It's a beautiful Art Deco building, built just before World War II, and has been described as architecturally the most important 20th century synagogue in England. The congregation was originally in Hope Place, just off Hope Street, in Liverpool city centre. But, after the First World War, Liverpool's Jews tended to move out of the city centre, and to the wealthier suburbs, like Childwall and Sefton Park. So in 1928 the Hope Place Congregation decided to move to Greenbank Drive, just off Smithdown Road and Ullet Road, and the new synagogue was opened in 1937. Incidentally, that old synagogue, on Hope Place, eventually became the Unity Theatre.

In its pomp the Greenbank Drive Synagogue was a beauty, but it was closed in 2008. It's a Grade II-listed building, so it's still standing, but the grounds are overgrown and derelict. The front gate hangs off its hinges, and the iron Star of David at the gate's centre is broken. If I had unlimited money, I'd love to sponsor its restoration, but the problem is there's no call for it. The Jewish community of my youth has evaporated.

When I was a kid there were about 8,000 Jews in Liverpool. But now there are about 1,200. The former Tory minister Edwina Currie, the former Attorney General Lord Goldsmith, the Harry Potter star Jason Isaacs… they all came from Liverpool's Jewish community and went on to great success in London. My pals, a lot of them, have gone to London too. Their kids went down to the Big Smoke first, and the parents have followed. It was a trickle at first. I can vaguely remember my cousin Andrea Berkoff emigrating to Melbourne and I'd completely forgotten about her after that until I met her at a funeral in Liverpool about five years ago. I immediately looked at her, 45-50 years on, and said, "You're Andrea, aren't you?" And we became best mates again. But Liverpool's Jewish community is an ageing community, and that trickle suddenly became a deluge. Watching the decline of the Jewish community has been like watching a game of Jenga, it collapsed almost overnight. Yet, just down the road, Manchester is one of the fastest-growing communities. That's quite a Hasidic community, though. They wouldn't like me much, a Jew who doesn't keep kosher. Especially when I've got a spare rib in my hand…

I remember as a kid there were many Jewish butchers in Liverpool. For instance, there were Bredski's on Penny Lane and Galkoff's on Pembroke Place. There was one, Mr Bloomberg, by the Feathers Hotel on Mount Pleasant, and I used to go in there with my mum. That was my mum's favourite butcher. I don't know why we went down there, but we would go on the bus, and he always used to have a stick of salami, a *Vursht* as he'd call it, which is Yiddish for the German *Wurst,* and he'd always say to me, "D'ya wanna piece of VOOSHT?!" Dead Scouse, he was, as they say in Liverpool. And I couldn't wait to get a piece of VOOSHT. I loved it.

The Vursht was a salami made by a company called Aaronovitch. It was beautiful. Aaronovitch is no more, and those Liverpool kosher butchers are no more. If you want a kosher butcher, you have to go to Manchester and Leeds. My dad's family lives around Leeds, and we'd go to Leeds and stock up at the butcher's, owned by a guy called Rosenhead. Mr Rosenhead was about 60, and he'd never seen the sea. He'd never set foot outside Leeds. His ambition was to go to Scarborough, but he'd never made it.

That was a very old-fashioned outlook, even then, which brings me back to my grandpa, Sidney. He and Edith lived around the corner from us. Their house may have been yards away geographically, but they lived a life that was light years away from our lifestyle.

This was a typically old-fashioned household. He would religiously return home in time for his evening meal of pickled beef and three boiled potatoes and a slice of bread and butter followed by two dessertspoons of ice cream - exactly as ordered in his strict diet. There was no variation whatsoever, to the extent that Edith would place his plate onto the table as Big Ben struck at 6pm prior to Radio 4 (or the Home Service as it would have been at the time) broadcasting the evening news.

Sidney had a business, SJ Green and Company. It was a rag trade in the old Taylor Street, off Scotland Road, and I was sent off during the school holidays, with a little briefcase and some kosher pickled beef sandwiches, and he would pay me to work there, just to get me off my mother's hands. And I got 25 shillings a week out of it, which was pretty good for a kid in those days. It soon went on sweets, because I loved sweets, especially Cadbury's chocolate. There was a window cleaners' department, and I'd sell the window cleaners chamois leathers through a little hatch window. His main business was serving ships with rags, great big bales of cloth - scrim - which would be sent off in lorries to shipping companies and they'd be transported all round the world. I used to be fascinated by his three-wheeled lorries with flat backs - Scammell Scarabs - and his whole business. But as he got older the business vanished, and Taylor Street was demolished, along with many of the roads off Scotland Road.

Grandpa Sidney was born on Brownlow Hill in 1894 and he had loads of brothers and sisters, a couple of whom went off to America in search of a better life. His younger sister was called Esther Greenberg, and she was the only relative of mine who was completely fluent in Yiddish. Yiddish and Scouse. My grandparents used to say things in Yiddish to each other when I was around if they didn't want me to understand, but once I started learning German their cover was blown.

Esther lived till she was 96. She was a comedienne and she used to go along to the Stapely Jewish old age home, on North Mossley Hill Road, where most of the audience were younger than her, and she would tell the rudest jokes you could ever imagine. They were filthy. She was an amazing woman. Sidney himself looked like Alfred Hitchcock, with his big round face. He used to imitate the way Hitchcock would say "Good evening" on his TV show when we went round there on a Saturday night. Grandma was religious but she was also really superstitious, and if ever, God forbid, there was a thunderstorm she'd say, "Hide ze cutlery! Knives and forks put away!" And she used to stand in the window of the study praying. She'd get the prayer book out. And they had a light in the hall, a great big tall thing, about 12 feet high, and my brother, Michael, who was an inveterate practical joker, would switch it on and off to make it look like lightning and he'd shout, "Look, grandma, thunderstorm!" And she would shriek, *"HEEYYY, OYYY, HEY!"*

It was when I was a child that I first learnt about diabetes, but it was a very shady knowledge. My mum, Hazel, and grandfather, Sidney, were diagnosed in the mid-60s. He was in his 60s, she was about 40. And they were ashamed of their diabetes, which these days would be considered unbelievable. But people really were not as upfront about it as today. The only other person I knew who had it was my mother's sister, Claire. Claire Fink was very eccentric and theatrical. And married to Colonel Gerald Fink, who'd you'd never dream was Jewish. He had a handlebar moustache, and loved hunting and fishing, and he was my grandfather's partner in the rag trade. Claire, on the other hand, was a journalist with the Liverpool Daily Post. She used to do a feature every week in the ladies' section called What's Inside Her Handbag? And she used to refer to celebrities every week and imagine what could be inside their handbags. I remember when she did an article on Princess Margaret, and all there was was gin. A packet of fags and a bottle of gin. If you've watched The Crown, you'd know just how spot-on Claire was.

Claire was diagnosed with her diabetes just after insulin treatment was developed in the late 20s, and she was forever being found in a comatose state in the city, because insulin was crude in those days. Even in the 60s, it was still animal insulin, but it had been refined. You could get short-term and long-term insulin. But back in Claire's day, it was what I can only describe as basic shit. And she would go into hypoglycaemic shock regularly. She was always ill with it.

On my dad's side, we had my Uncle George, who lived with his sister, Aunt Becky. We would visit them in Leeds, along with other members of the extended family, and at some point in the evening, a card game would start. This would involve the uncles and the cousins, and would carry on until about 1am, or until I'd reminded my dad that I had school in the morning. George used to take our family to the Motor Show in Earls Court every year. We'd go there for half-term, and he'd take us to a restaurant called the Roman Room in Brompton Street. All the waiters and waitresses were dressed as Romans, and I had chicken in a basket, in which the basket was made of chips. That was my favourite meal, oh, the sophistication! But going down to Earls Court was even more magical because George would get us through the queues and we would never have to wait.

If Judaism was my childhood's official religion, the religion I followed most fervently also met for worship on Saturdays, mostly at Goodison Park. I became an Evertonian by virtue of two reasons. The first was the influence of Harvey Harrison. Harvey was my brother Michael's best friend, and he was a mad Evertonian. Some would say that's the only sort of Evertonian. I hero-worshipped Harvey Harrison. If he'd said, "Support Man United," I would have done. But he supported Everton, so if anybody asked me who I supported, it was Everton. In fact, before I even went to Goodison for the first time, we were moving from the surgery on Storrsdale Road to the new house, and we had carpets being fitted. I was chatting to the carpet-fitter and I was only six years old, and he said, "Ey, lad, who do yer support?"

I squeaked, "Everton!"

He said, "Don't do it, they'll break yer bloody heart." He wasn't wrong. So Harvey Harrison sowed the seeds. I like to say I was radicalised by Harvey.

But what really sealed the deal was my first proper match. I remember it like it was yesterday. I can still recite the team formation. It was on 9 January 1965, against Sheffield Wednesday in the FA Cup. My dad had a surgery in Roscommon Street, near Goodison, on Saturday mornings, and that day a patient came in. He said, "'Ey, doc, I've got two tickets to Everton, and I can't go cos me wife's not well. Would you like them for you and your lad?" So, my dad came home with two tickets, and he said, "Do you want to go and see Everton?" And it took a micro-second for me to decide…

We were in the Upper Bullens Road stand, and every time we got a corner, which was about once every hour - typical Everton - everybody would bang their feet on the floor, and I had to stand up to bang my feet because I was so little and my feet dangled off the seat. It was a 2-2 draw, and that was it. I was an Evertonian for life. I found the programme for that game 10 years ago. I've got it framed in my house.

The replay was the following Tuesday at Hillsborough and, of course, I was too young to be going to the match, especially an away game in Sheffield. And the results used to come on the BBC Light Programme - which is Radio 2 now - at five to 10. And my mum was making the beds while my dad was out playing bridge, and the results came on. "Here are tonight's football results, FA Cup Third Round Replay, blah-de-blah-de-blah, Sheffield Wednesday 0 Everton 3," and I jumped on the bed, bouncing up and down, and my mum gave me such a whack. "Get off my bed!" I think it was my first experience of football hooliganism.

The following year, Uncle George took me to Amsterdam for my bar mitzvah present, and he said, "I'm taking you to Amsterdam for the motor show." Obviously, I was delighted - I loved our trips to Earls Court, and this was going to be even better. But when we got there, it turned out to be a commercial motor show, full of tractors and lorries, and I was bored out of my skull. He had an agent called Mr Mulder, and Mrs Mulder used to take me on day trips every day. It was the week before Everton in the FA Cup in 1966, and I was desperate to get back. I didn't have tickets, I was too young, but on Cup Final Day, I wanted to watch my heroes, and George had taken me to the seaside for the day. And the last thing he wanted to do was watch bloody football. He was only interested in wrestling, like my dad. Not with my dad, but like my dad, although the two of them did have a wrestle occasionally. They were both very temperamental. It took till about quarter to four to find a hotel with a telly in where I could watch the second half of the cup final, and I watched Mike Trebilcock and Derek Temple winning the cup for us. So I was on a high, and Uncle George said to me, "Do you want to stay on another week?"

I said, "No! I want to be in Mossley Hill to see the team coming back on an open-top bus!" So that curtailed the trip to what should have been a fantastic Motor Show, and which turned out to be the most boring instead. I've never seen anything like it, just truck after truck. God, I went to see Ferraris and all I saw were Scammels. I could have done that at my grandfather's factory and saved Uncle George a fortune.

The year after that, I went back to northern Europe and had a much better time. When I had been 11, I had made what in retrospect was one of the most significant decisions of my life. I had to make a choice at school between geography and history or German, which was a ridiculously terrible choice, because I like geography… I like the weather. I was fascinated by the weather. All I did during geography lessons was analyse weather maps. I could study them forever. But I had to give up geography, because I was desperate to do languages. However, that choice opened up the world to me in a way that geography never could. It was to give me the confidence I needed after my diagnosis. And it would introduce me to one of my closest friends.

At first, I was disastrous at German - I was in detention every night - but eventually, I began to get the hang of it. In the Lent term we had the opportunity of going to Germany on an exchange trip - three weeks in Germany and your partner, whoever he may be, would come back to Liverpool in the summer for three weeks.

So we applied around Christmas time, and then one Saturday morning we received information from a company in Finland which was sorting out the exchanges, with details of this guy in Germany called Ulrich Fuchs. Fuchs means Fox, although a lot of people assumed it meant something else... And Ulrich looked like a real blond, blue-eyed, Aryan German. This filled me with horror. At the time, I was 13, going on 14, and my parents said, "You can only go if another boy from your class goes to the same village." So this guy from my class, Stephen Coy, and I were paired up with two Ulrichs - Ulrich Fuchs and Stephen's partner Ulrich Gockel. The only similarity between them was their names. The two Ulrichs knew each other, but my Ulrich hated the other because he was a swot. But he was friendly enough.

We'd had an exciting train journey across Europe starting off at Lime Street, going down to Victoria, where we were meeting up with other schools, and then crossing the Channel, ending up on the train to Mainz. I didn't know anybody from the other schools, there were probably about two or three hundred, but we didn't really get to know anybody. I do remember there was one very pretty young lady, but she was too pretty and tall for me. I was only about 4ft 6ins, a little tiny boy and Uli was about 6ft. So the discrepancy between us was amazing.

We arrived at Mainz and Uli Gockel's father picked us up. And in the back of the car were my Uli, Stephen and Uli Gockel and they took us to our house in Bad Wildungen where the first thing we did when we arrived was kick a football around, but then I collapsed in a heap.

I'll always remember being rather Jewish and they were religiously Catholic. They took me to my room, and I screamed in horror when I saw a crucifix over the bed. And, of course, because I was a little boy, I was very homesick immediately. My parents would send me a box of chocolates - the Crunchies and Mars Bars that little did I know a year later would be completely vetoed.

We didn't see much of Uli Gockel except when riding to school on bikes. Stephen and I were at school with our exchange partners for three weeks and we'd ride there every day, but Gockel had an artificial leg and he couldn't understand why we were having such a struggle getting up the hill on the bikes. I was at his house once, looking under the stairs in the cloakroom, and found all different sizes of false legs. He must have kept them as he grew up. Lord knows what he was planning to do with them.

One night, my Uli and I were invited round for dinner. Now, Uli Gockel's father was a very hospitable guy, friendly, like his son. He took us on trips to the east-west border and various other attractions, and he was the kindest man you could wish to meet. Before dinner, he said, "I know you're Jewish and you don't eat pork, but can you eat chicken?"

I said, "That's fine. Thanks very much." It was a lovely dinner, and halfway through, I asked, "Could I use your toilet, please?" And he said, "Yes, of course." I didn't speak any English, so I was using broken German. My Uli was perfect in English. So I went upstairs, walked down the corridor to the toilet, and, to my absolute amazement and horror, there was a photograph of Herr Gockel in full Nazi uniform.

Although I was little, I wasn't shy, and I went downstairs and said, "Herr Gockel, can you explain that photograph on the landing? You know, that interesting photograph…?" And he said to me, "Well, I must tell you about that. In about 1930, we were sitting in the lounge, listening to the radio, and there was a knock on the door and there were two men from the National Socialist Party and they asked us whether we'd be interested in joining their party. And we said no. No interest whatsoever. Thank you.

"He said, 'Well, I'll leave you some literature. I will come back next week and see if you've changed your mind.' Anyway, they came back the following week. And we said we were not interested. Thank you. They said, 'Well, we have to tell you that we will come to power within a couple of years. And when we do we will take your business from you and you'll be in grave danger.' So what could we do?" I accepted that totally, and that was done.

It wasn't until about 2005 that one morning, very early, I woke up and nudged my wife and said, "The bloody bastard! If he's so ashamed, why's he got the photograph on display?" It took me nearly 40 years to work that out, which shows how stupid I am and how gullible people were in those days, but he was an extremely friendly bloke.

It was a fascinating trip. People were just so nice, but things were different in those days. We were there on Good Friday and we used to play table tennis in the apartment above us, which belonged to a Herr Fischer. We were bored, because in West Germany on Good Friday there was no television and there was no radio. Herr Fischer was just playing opera all day long. We were bored out of our skulls, so we went up and knocked on his door and asked if we could play table tennis, and he said, "It's Good Friday! Don't you know the world doesn't exist on Good Friday?" It was so religious. It was unbelievable. So we just went off and played football on our own.

And, so, that was the life that was turned upside down, the life of a happy, normal kid from south Liverpool, who loved sweets so much that even the football team he followed was nicknamed "the Toffees". But, during the winter of 1967-68, when I was 14, I developed a run of colds and infections, and my energy levels were dropping dramatically whenever I played football. Something was very wrong...

2
My Hero Heinz

In the winter of 1967-68, my dream of emulating my Everton foot-balling heroes was vanishing before my very eyes.

For 10 minutes, I'd be playing like Alan Ball, Colin Harvey, and Howard Kendall combined, and then my energy levels would collapse. I'd normally be playing in Calderstones Park, just over the road from my house, and I'd feel awful, and the thirst would start. So I'd go home and have a bowl of cornflakes with loads of sugar, or eat a Crunchie bar, or drink lemonade. And this would just make my situation worse, by increasing my already high blood sugar level, even though for a few minutes I felt reinvigorated.

Before this, I'd been aware something was wrong. We had a party at home, and I spoke to my dad. I'd seen diabetes in my mum and my grandpa Sidney, and I told my dad, "You know, I'm sure I'm becoming diabetic. I'm getting very thirsty." And he dismissed my concerns. But I'd clearly put a marker at the back of his mind.

But again in mid-January 1968 I was off school with another cold, and I was suffering the most awful, unquenchable thirst. By the time my father came home from surgery, I was drinking my fourth cup of tea. When he witnessed me pouring my fifth cup, he pulled his glasses down and stared at me before remarking that I was drinking rather a lot.

I told him I just couldn't control my thirst and I felt rotten. The thought of diabetes was a great fear for me. I had seen how being diabetic had affected my mother and grandfather, as well as my

Aunt Claire. My mum and grandpa Sidney were diagnosed within four years of each other and their diagnoses had upset them greatly. They never liked to discuss diabetes, and it was a taboo topic in our household despite how large it loomed.

My dad put his glasses back on and immediately drove to the local pharmacy for some home urine-testing strips. It became clear that the reading of sugar content was almost off the scale. He was on the phone within seconds and an appointment was made for the following Monday, 16 January 1968, with Dr Heinz Fuld.

Much of this book is about my heroes, the people who have inspired me through my struggle with diabetes, the people who have lifted me up when I've felt low and put me back on the right path. Heinz Fuld is, perhaps, the greatest of those heroes. I would not be here today without him.

I first encountered him a couple of years earlier. We had a dog, Rusty, a boxer, who we all loved. My brother Michael was asthmatic and struggling, and his specialist, Dr Ansell, told him, "You're allergic to the dog. Get rid of the dog." So we had to put Rusty in kennels the next day. It was heartbreaking. But Michael's symptoms did not improve. My dad asked for a second opinion, from Dr Fuld, who he knew professionally. Dr Fuld came around and examined him. He was a tall, imposing, angular man, with half-moon spectacles, extremely Teutonic. He peered at Michael, then said, "Hmm, you all miss the dog and the dog misses you. Get him home." We didn't need to be told twice and we were reunited with our beloved Rusty. It turned out that Michael was allergic to horses, not dogs.

I will never forget Dr Fuld's surgery. The stone floors and lack of soft furnishings gave 69 Rodney Street, near to Liverpool's Anglican cathedral, a very Germanic appearance which would not have looked out of place in a World War II film set in Gestapo headquarters.

But this was ironic. Heinz Fuld was as far from a Nazi as you could possibly get. A Christian of Jewish descent, he escaped from Germany in the early 30s, as the Nazis started to take over public life in his home country. He had attended Hitler's rallies along with a friend as an observer, and been attacked when he refused to stand and applaud.

He had received his medical doctorate from Heidelberg in 1931, and went to work in Freiburg, but in May 1933, a violent anti-se-mitic manifesto - "Against the Un-German Spirit" - was displayed at Freiburg University. Wilhelm von Mollendorf, Professor of Anatomy, ordered the removal of the posters from the premises of the university, and was immediately sacked. Every Jewish doctor at the university hospital was given 24 hours to leave.

Dr Fuld went to Berlin to visit Professor Unger, the father of one of his friends from his student years. According to Fuld's unpub-lished memoirs, which were kindly loaned to me by his daughter, Susan Evans:

"Professor Unger was well informed politically. He advised me to leave Germany as soon as possible and suggested I should move to Edin-burgh where I had a chance to requalify within a year, in contrast to all universities in England, which insisted on a two-year study."

Fuld went to Edinburgh, without being able to speak a word of English on arrival, and qualified, before eventually settling in gen-eral practice in Liverpool. Professor Unger, who was Jewish him-self, was forced to stay, and ended his own life in 1939 by driving his Mercedes at high speed against a stone wall.

Dr Fuld had been writing to his sister and brother-in-law in Munich and to his parents in Mannheim urging them to leave. But his father took his own life. In the end, Fuld was able to secure the release of his sick mother from Germany for £2,000, equivalent to around £130,000 today.

Fuld himself, like my father, joined the British armed forces, and he became a major in the Royal Medical Army Corps. Following the end of the war in Europe, he was one of the first doctors to enter Bergen-Belsen concentration camp upon its liberation. After he was demobbed, he joined Sefton General Hospital on Smith-down Road, Liverpool, as a physician, with his private practice at

69 Rodney Street, which is where I was taken by my mother on that fateful day.

Heinz Fuld may have looked terrifying in a Teutonic way, but as a person he was anything but. He had a very dry sense of humour but also a heart of gold. He asked me about my symptoms and observed me. I had been hanging on to the hope that my problem was a condition called glycosuria, from which my Uncle George - who also had sugar in his water - had suffered, but Dr Fuld firmly, but kindly, dismissed that.

Then he lifted the receiver of the phone on his desk, called Sefton General Hospital, and spoke those life-changing words: "I wish to reserve a bed for Laurence Lee, diabetic." I was diabetic, and at the tender age of 14 it felt like the end of the world.

My first thought was that I would never be able to eat Cadbury's chocolate ever again.

My second thought was about how I could possibly handle injecting myself, given my dread of needles

But my biggest fear was that I may not be well enough to watch my beloved Everton Football Club.

I can't imagine what my poor mother must have thought. It must have been awful for her, because she felt guilty: one, because I had inherited it from her, and two, because it was such a taboo illness. If she'd realised that I would be openly shouting it from the rooftops, and writing a book about it many years later, I like to think she'd have been proud, rather than guilty. It seems silly for her to feel guilty about it, but I understand how she must have felt because I was so relieved that I haven't passed it on to my own daughters.

But back to Dr Fuld, and my first consultation. He took a blood test to see how high my blood sugar level was. His humour was evident when, having completed his blood-letting exercise, he told me to keep my arm above my head for three weeks. In those days, the maximum reading should have been 180. My first reading was 325. He said, "Right, no carbohydrates for you. You will have just meat, fish, and eggs, and you will test your blood again in two days."

His plan was to starve me of carbohydrates for the rest of the week to see how far my readings fell. I was allowed to eat as much protein as I liked, but under no circumstances was I permitted to touch sweets, especially my beloved Cadbury's chocolate.

Lo and behold, my readings, which started out around three times the normal level, fell to 225 within a couple of days, and by the Friday my blood sugar reading was still too high but was reducing without insulin, which would not be used on me till I was admitted to hospital on Sunday, 21 January, and I must admit I felt a little bit better, but far from 100 per cent.

I was dreading the idea of being hospitalised for up to two weeks, which was the norm in those days. They called it standardisation.

I would initially be on Dr Fuld's regime of three soluble (quick-acting) insulin injections daily and a fixed diet of 180g of carbohydrates, split into three main meals, plus afternoon and late evening snacks. For a boy of my age, 180g of carbohydrates was beyond comprehension, but I got hold of what was called an exchange list which taught me very quickly that there was actually nothing that I couldn't eat as long as I kept within my limit. Unfortunately I got off to a very bad start. Fearing that I had eaten my last ever piece of chocolate, I foolishly gave myself a parting treat just before I left home for hospital in the form of a Cadbury's Creme Egg. It was delicious and I thought nobody would ever find out. How wrong I was.

Into my room walked my hero Heinz Fuld at around 6pm, and he said, "Have you something to tell me, young man?" I played dumb and said I had no idea what he meant.

"Your blood sugar tonight is now higher than last week when we first met."

The game was up and he made it quite clear that this stupidity had to stop and my diet of 180g of carbohydrates was to be strictly adhered to.

That wasn't my only act of self-sabotage in those 10 days, however. I was a physically immature 14-year-old, with a face as smooth as a snooker ball. Even so, I decided that I would need to shave while I was in hospital. Really, regular shaving would be a year away, but I took a shaver into hospital with me, in the form of a Schick razor blade.

In order to change the blade, you had to shove it into a little gadget which would "inject" the blade into the shaver. You had to be really careful, though, and make sure your finger was nowhere near the blade as it shot into place. I think you've read enough of this book so far to guess what happened next…

So, within five minutes of arriving in my hospital room – Room 17 – I was in casualty because I'd nearly chopped my finger off. This, combined with the Creme Egg fiasco, prompted Dr Fuld practically to tie me to the bed until the insulin kicked in…

After the insulin took effect, however, Dr Fuld made it quite clear that there would be no sitting around in my room and that I was to remain active as soon as I felt stronger. This only took a couple of days. My fear of needles disappeared as soon as the beneficial effects of insulin took hold, starting with the disappearance, thank heavens, of my dreadful thirst.

And at that point I was able to enjoy my afternoon treat. Each afternoon I was treated to my afternoon snack, which consisted of two Jacob's Cream Crackers and a smidgeon of butter. I particularly enjoyed these for a very strange reason. At Liverpool College, during every tasteless lunch to which we were subjected on a daily basis, I would look jealously towards the prefects' table, where they would tuck into cheese and crackers, while we had some revolting semolina or bread and butter pudding. I knew I would never reach prefect status because I wasn't a rugby player, a creep, or a school bully, so when I was offered daily crackers in hospital I was delighted.

But after a few days, they became a little bit bland, and that's when my lovely mum Hazel discovered a very tasty diabetic jam (a very rare event) made by Frank Cooper. To my delight she brought in a small jar of this very tasty preserve for me to try, like the small jars of jam available in hotels. This was fantastic, and I poured as much jam as I could onto my two little crackers, which, incidentally, consisted of 5g of carbohydrate each, until it was about six inches high.

As I was munching away at this delightful concoction, I was avidly reading the jar to check up on the contents. It was so sweet tasting that I couldn't believe that it didn't contain any actual sugar. It actually contained a sweetening agent called sorbitol and, as I was devouring this newly discovered treat, I noticed a warning on the jar relating to maximum daily intake.

Oh, my God! I had exceeded it fourfold and, no sooner had I finished reading the warning, I immediately began to suffer the effects of excessive intake. I had never been a world champion sprinter, but I swear that I broke the indoor record over the distance between Room 17 and the very welcoming toilet down the seemingly never-ending corridor.

That overindulgence with Frank Cooper cost me two extra days in hospital, but at least it proved that I was recovering my athletic prowess.

Having been firmly put in my place and confined to quarters by Dr Fuld, I set about contemplating my situation and wondered what lay ahead. I was comforted by the 60s gramophone my parents had installed, and relaxed to my favourite music of the time especially The Beatles' *Magical Mystery Tour* album and lots of soul especially the Four Tops and the Temptations, Motown acts who were adored by my older brother, Michael. My reading material consisted of football magazines and a big Everton poster that the nurses allowed me to pin onto the wall.

Unfortunately, my stay in hospital was hardly a cakewalk, if you'll excuse the expression. My supportive school, Liverpool College, had sent textbooks and homework for me to complete, but, more importantly, I needed to get to the bottom of what caused diabetes and any other information I could get my hands on.

Thanks to my dad's medical experience I had access to plenty of literature relating to diabetes which explained how a breakdown in the pancreas, in particular the islets of Langerhans, resulted in a failure to produce insulin either totally or partially.

Insulin is a crucial hormone in breaking down sugars into energy - like a carburettor in a car. Without insulin the sugar levels rise to the extent that excess sugar flows into the urine and that's how my condition was detected.

During my time in hospital I had plenty of time to worry about what the future held for me. None of my school contemporaries were diabetic. Diabetes, although by no means rare, was nowhere near as common as it is today, particularly Type 2 late onset/obesity-induced diabetes, so I had nobody of my age to turn to for advice.

On the other hand, I realised that I would be able to use my condition as a perfect excuse for missing rugby and other onerous activities that I didn't fancy three times a week.

I only had my grandfather and my mother to talk to, but, being very old school, they were of no use scientifically, although their love and support were priceless.

During my stay in hospital I began to set myself targets, including how soon I could get back to watching my beloved Everton. The fifth round of the FA Cup was due to take place at home to Tranmere Rovers on 9 March, and I made that match my prime target. I was determined that neither wild horses nor diabetes would keep me away from watching my heroes, even if I'd only been out of hospital for five weeks.

I always went to the match with my dad who, although originally from Yorkshire, had become an avid Evertonian because of me. This would be my first match post-hospital and would be another step towards normality of life.

But it would never be completely normal. My life was changed forever that winter. Even in 1968, while I found myself in a situation far more desirable than life would be in the 20s, things were far from easy for me, having to adapt to a life of daily injections and a strict diet or regime of 180g of carbohydrates to be taken at fairly exact times.

Every day, even now, I thank my lucky stars that I wasn't around in the early 20th century or even earlier, when the choice open to a diabetic patient was either to try and survive on an almost calorie-free diet and slowly waste away, or (as the *Reader's Digest* German edition article on the discovery of insulin stated) eat well today and die tomorrow. Although I was lucky enough to become a diabetic in the late 60s, please don't think for one moment that I was in for an easy ride for many years to come. I used to lie awake in hospital worrying about how I would cope in the outside world with diabetes. I worried about how I would handle injections, which Dr Fuld had reduced to twice-daily in time for my return home.

I was prescribed a mixture of quick-acting soluble insulin and a slower-acting type called isophane, which in my early years was in animal form.

When I entered Sefton General Hospital I weighed in at 6st 10lb and was bordering on being emaciated. Within 10 days I had recovered to 8st 4lb. Gradually, we had got my treatment right, and, much to the relief of the marvellous staff of Sefton General, I was discharged. I came out of hospital feeling better, because my sugars were normal. But physically I was in second gear. I would have to learn to manage my condition and get better. Heinz Fuld had given me a second chance, it was up to me now to take it.

3
Back To School

When I left hospital in February 1968, I decided I wasn't going to be a boring diabetic. To me, the epitome of a boring diabetic was my beloved grandfather, Sidney. He, as I said, had exactly the same meal every single night - two slices of pickled beef, three boiled potatoes, two slices of very thin Warburton's bread - and my grandmother Edith would put it on the table as Big Ben struck six, or his whole world would implode. This wasn't just because he was an austere creature of habit. It was his way of controlling the amount of carbohydrates he consumed. It was his way of controlling his diabetes.

I was never going to live that way. On leaving hospital, I was given an exchange list, a sacred document which allowed me to live my best life. It showed me exactly what I could eat. I was allowed 6.5oz of carbohydrates a day, made up of 2oz at breakfast, 1oz at lunch, 2oz at dinner, and the odd ounce here or there for snacks. And this exchange list told me what constituted 1oz of carbs. So I knew, for example, that 1oz could be two-thirds of an ounce of bread. Or, joy of joys, the same amount of Cadbury's Dairy Milk chocolate, because Cadbury's Dairy Milk had exactly the same sugar content as bread. One of my biggest fears on being diagnosed diabetic was that I would never be able to eat Cadbury's chocolate, and now I could fill my boots. Well, within reason. So, instead of having a piece of bread, I'd have a chunk of chocolate. It psychologically boosted me to know I could eat those things.

Do you have any idea what 3oz of chips looks like? No, neither did I, especially at first. And so, whenever I went out for a meal, I'd have to take along my trusty scales. My parents had bought me a small set when I left hospital, and my mum would carry them in her handbag. These would enable me to weigh all my carbohydrates, such as my beloved chips. I even took my scales into cafés and restaurants, which always raised a few eyebrows, especially when once we were on holiday to North Wales. Onlookers probably thought a drugs deal was underway, although my dear parents hardly looked like drug barons. I got to the stage within six months where I could look at a plate of food and know exactly the carbohydrate content of everything on it, mashed potatoes, boiled potatoes, chips, a glass of milk with it, a couple of slices of bread which had been weighed, and that would make up my quota. So I was a dab hand… I would go looking at other people's plates and think, "Ooh, he's got one and a half ounces of carbohydrate. Big fat pig, he's got three ounces," when I could only have half that. I became neurotic and a nerd about weighing food.

I wasn't quite ready for school when I left hospital. It had been agreed with Liverpool College that I would stay off until Easter to enable me to acclimatise to everyday life as an insulin-dependant diabetic. Luckily, the year before, at the age of 14, I had passed three O Levels, in French, German, and Maths. But I didn't pass the other five I had taken. I was so frightened that my dad would shout at me. So when the results came out, I hid next door, at the house of my friend Stuart Miller. Dad knocked at the door, and I was terrified, convinced he was going to come and belt me.

But he said, "I am absolutely delighted with the fact that you managed to get three O Levels at the age of 14. It's incredible. And here's a little present for you." He reached into his pocket and pulled out two tickets for Everton v Wolves that afternoon. And off we went to Goodison. The legendary Derek Dougan was playing for Wolves that day, but we won 4-2, so it was a great day. I'm a big fan of the book *Fever Pitch*, by Nick Hornby. It really speaks to me, because everything in the hero's life revolves around football. And everything I do ties back to "I know what I was doing then, because they were playing." I can remember every match.

So my dad was delighted, and, funnily enough, the only time I ever got any kind of prize after an exam was after I'd failed, because I still looked upon this as failure, as I'd passed just three out of eight O Levels, even though I was only 14. So the school, instead of putting me in the dunces' reform class, said, "Look, Lee, you were stupid to take them at that age. You repeat the year." Or words to that effect. So I was able to stay in the A class, and it would turn out that missing a whole term was not a disaster as I'd merely be going over old ground.

But, before I went back to school, I had to keep my hospital promise to myself, and go to see the Blues play Tranmere Rovers in the FA Cup Fifth Round. The match against Tranmere wasn't a classic, but we won 2-0, my now dear friend Joe Royle scored, and it was another milestone for me, showing me that not everything in my life had to change. Accompanying me and my dad that day was my young next-door neighbour Stuart Miller, who was 13 years old at the time. Stuart, who was prepared to shelter me from the wrath of my dad, turned gamekeeper years later, and now sits as a criminal district judge having, like me, been a criminal lawyer for over 30 years. I just prayed that Everton could win a couple more cup games and make it to Wembley for the FA Cup Final. I felt that I'd been through the mill, and the least I deserved was my first ever walk down Wembley Way.

When I went back to school, I had to get used to my new status quo. At first, my dad would inject me, twice a day. The thought of injecting myself was frightening. They weren't exactly great big hypodermic needles, like the sort of epidural needle that women have during labour, but they were still a quarter of an inch long, which is quite a lot to stick into your leg when you're a kid. You would assume my dad would have been the King of Injections. After all, during the war, he'd done 20,000 at a time. But in the mornings, before school, he was half-asleep, and I think he injected the wall twice. He had clearly lost his talent.

So, fairly soon after I returned to school, I said to him, "Look, I'm going to have to learn to do this myself." It was a matter of self-preservation. And I couldn't have him coming around when I was married for 30 years, knocking on the door every morning to say, "Excuse me, Mrs. Lee, can I inject your husband, please?" So I learnt to do it myself, and it became easier, though it was never fun. I'd inject myself in the thigh rather than the stomach, which was recommended. You could say I didn't have the stomach for it. The tissue in my thigh became spongy after a while. I would have to draw up two different types of insulin - slow-acting and quick-acting - and mix them in the syringe. It would take three or four minutes, whereas now it takes seconds. We diabetics were on this animal insulin and, looking back, it was awful. I felt in second gear and that was normal to me. It was only when they finally brought in human insulin in the 70s that I changed over. I was prescribed bovine insulin - ox insulin. Porcine insulin - pig insulin - was also available, but I never had that. I would have had it if I had needed to, even though I was Jewish, because my religion taught me that it would have been a greater sin not to use pig insulin if it made you better. Bovine insulin was very crude, and the quick-acting variety really was quick acting. Ten minutes after taking it, you could feel your blood sugar going down. The long-acting variety had peaks of four hours, which mean that if you didn't eat on time, you'd risk a terrible hypoglycaemic episode.

Now, like my dad so many times in those late-night card games in Leeds, I felt I'd been dealt a bloody awful hand when I was diagnosed. I was going to be diabetic for the rest of my life. But, when life serves you a lemon, you make lemonade, and I found ways to take advantage of my condition. Well, it was only fair...

For starters, when I restarted at Liverpool College, I was able to con the school into allowing me to go home for lunch. No more disgusting bowls of semolina or bread-and-butter pudding. No more gazing at the prefects with jealousy as they gnawed on their cheese and crackers. My dear dad would pick me up after his surgery at 12.30ish and I'd go home and enjoy mum's food. I could weigh my chips or bread and butter without the public glaring at me. I'd always try to get back to school early enough to join in the daily playground football kickaround. I would be invited to be the late super sub and even score the winner, when I would be mobbed as if I'd won the Cup Final. My self-confidence soon began to return.

Even better, my diabetes got me sympathy. Being the only diabetic in the school made it easy for me to skive off rugby and athletics. Nobody in authority would ever question me if I claimed not to feel up to doing strenuous sport.

It was all going swimmingly until another pupil, who I'll call Humphries, became diabetic in 1969. He was captain of the school athletics team prior to diagnosis. To my horror, he was back to pre-diabetes levels of fitness within weeks. My cover had been blown and I was summoned to the headmaster's study.

Mr Collinson, our fearsome headmaster, wanted to know how Humphries was back to full strength within weeks of becoming diabetic, whereas I was only able to dip my toe into the world of strenuous sport despite the passing of over a year.

I took a breath, and mustered the powers of persuasion that would serve me well in my future career as a criminal solicitor. "Well, sir," I said, "what you have to understand is that all diabetics are different." The headmaster's response still rings in my ears.

"That, Lee," he barked, "is patently obvious."

I was told in no uncertain terms that I was to report for rugby practice the next day. My ploy was over thanks to that traitor Humphries. Fortunately, Mr Collinson hadn't cottoned on that I wasn't on any roll calls. However, I was always good at running. I wasn't on the 100 metres team, but I could get to a reasonable standard. And so, when the athletics season started, Lee would occasionally make an appearance.

The day of my diagnosis, 16 January, may have been the low

point of my year and maybe my life so far. Four months later, on 18 May 1968, I cried with emotion as my dad and I realised our dream and together (with a Mars bar in my pocket) walked down Wembley Way to watch our Everton heroes play against West Bromwich Albion in the FA Cup Final.

Dad had a twin, Maurice - Uncle Mot - who was a director of Kettering Town FC, and he sold us their complete allocation of two tickets at the extortionate price of £2 each. We strutted down Wembley Way, feeling very optimistic as we'd beaten West Brom 6-2 a few weeks earlier. Sadly, the walk back up Wembley Way was not so joyous, as we lost 1-0 in extra time, and my heart was broken by a Jeff Astle thunderbolt. At least I had achieved one major dream...

That summer, I retook my O Levels, and I passed the same three subjects plus four more, so no damage was done, and I could proceed to A Levels, when I would take French, German, and English, and aim to study law at whichever university I could. People often wonder why I chose law - as do I after a bad day in court - especially as my father was a doctor. Why didn't I go into medicine? After all, I'd have been a dab hand at administering injections...

The fact is, I'd wanted to go into medicine, but I couldn't do science to save my life, or anybody else's. I nearly blew up the school lab once, trying to light a Bunsen burner, forgetting to put the cord in and just lighting the gas at the tap. I was a disaster at sciences. I was good at maths, though. My dad was very good at mental arithmetic and I've inherited that. It's handy for working out VAT and bills and things. Also, I wasn't keen on the sight of blood, which doesn't help with a career in the medical profession. If I'd have been a doctor, there'd have been a sign in the waiting room saying, "No blood cases, please."

But I inherited a facility for languages from my mum. She was arty and good at French, and, above all, a poetess, who used to bombard the BBC Radio Merseyside presenter Roger Phillips with her compositions. And she was a tremendous bullshitter, which I've inherited too. Also, my Aunt Beck and Uncle Alec in Leeds had a son, Malcolm Sorkin, who became the top criminal lawyer in the West Riding of Yorkshire, and I looked up to him. I called him Uncle Malcolm, even though he was my cousin. The plan was that he, my brother Michael, and I would go into law practice together. But that wasn't to be. While I was finding my feet, in March 1974, Malcolm and his wife, Ruth, were tragically killed when Turkish Airlines Flight 981 crashed outside Paris, taking the lives of all 346 people on board. Malcolm and Ruth were in their early forties, and they left two young children, aged just ten and six. And the following year, we were to lose Michael too.

But back to 1968, and in the space of a few months, I'd made it to football matches, gone back to school, and passed my exams. That year may not have been so bad after all. It wasn't all plain sailing, though. People had an ignorant view of diabetics, which, I'm sure, was mostly to blame for the shame my poor mum and grandfather felt about our shared condition. When we visited my mum's friend's house, she was giving out sweets to the kids there. She said, "John, would you like a piece of chocolate? Alan, would you like a piece of chocolate?" Then, when she got to me, she said, "No, Laurence, you can't have chocolate," and snatched it away. Of course I felt mortified, as if there were a prejudice against me. She wasn't the only one. People would often say to me, "Why! You can't have sugar!" There was a myth that a diabetic can't eat sugar.

I'd reply, "Well, if I can't eat sugar, you'd better book my funeral pretty quick, because a car needs petrol, and, beforehand, it wasn't converting it into energy. I've got a carburettor now, thanks, in the form of insulin." But you'd try to explain that to someone, and ignorance was hard to shift. After all, there weren't many of us around.

The pioneering diabetes survivor Alan Nabarro, who we'll meet in the next chapter, talked about the prejudice he got from weighing his food or going into the toilet for an injection as a child. I couldn't give two hoots about it now, I'd laugh my socks off. But to a kid in his early teens, that would be devastating. If you were delicate, it could give you a nervous breakdown. You'd hide away…

There are many adjectives people would use to describe me. I doubt "delicate" would be among them. I'd never hide away my diabetes. If anything, I was proud of it. It was standard for my friends to say, "You going for your jab now?" And, because I was managing it so well, my mum felt confident and happier, and I think her guilt trip diminished, quite rightly so. But my grandfather Sidney never changed his ways, sticking with his two slices of pickled beef every night.

I carried on eating sweets, but they were all accounted for. Life became a balancing act. The motto of the British Diabetic Association was "Balance" and you really did have to balance. But the vast majority of diabetics didn't balance at all, and those were the ones who had ridiculously high blood sugar and would go on to get complications. At that time, you'd hear of people with serious eye damage, limb wasting, lack of circulation leading to lost legs, and all sorts of complaints, and I was determined that wouldn't happen to me. But I was equally determined that I would live as normal a life as possible. Now that's balance.

After my O Levels in 1968, my focus shifted to my A Levels in 1970. I decided to do French, English, and German, with my main target being to get into Liverpool University. And my good friend Ulrich Fuchs helped my German so much. Uli had come to Liverpool in the summer before I went into hospital, and he became close to my brother, Michael, because he was nearer Michael's age. He was his size, too, and they got on like a house on fire. But he always looked after me, he was like my second big brother. At that time I didn't eat a lot. I was a very little boy and he'd say, "Come on, eat some more potatoes." I'd say, "No, I don't want to."

He'd say, "Come on, do it for Everton." And of course then I'd do it. He remains one of my dearest friends.

But in 1969, I was beginning to worry about three-hour exams. And I did an exam called Use of English, which should have been called Useless English, because I was a disaster. Halfway through the exam, I started getting nervous because I was behind and my handwriting just seized up, so I thought I had low blood sugar. So the invigilators gave me sugary water, and I failed the exam - I just couldn't complete it. I went home and my blood sugar was sky high. Looking back, I think the adrenaline flowed and my body couldn't handle it. But by the time 1970 came around, it was easy, because I'd read so much French and German literature. The French and German books on my A Level syllabus were inspiring, especially *Le Grand Meaulnes* by Alain-Fournier. This book has inspired me throughout my life, because it showed me that if I relentlessly pursued my dreams as the hero Meaulnes did, no aspiration would be impossible. At the other end of the spectrum, I devoured the *Reader's Digest* in German, where I learned so much about diabetes - and I learned incredible words, like the German for "stomach juices". I'm not sure how often this extensive vocabulary would have come in handy for tourists, but you should never knock learning. In any case, thanks to Uli and the *Reader's Digest,* I sailed through my German. And, a couple of years later, I'd put that German to good use...

I applied for various universities - Liverpool, Manchester, Leeds, all places I knew well - and last on my UCCA list was Warwick University. Most of them summarily rejected me because of my age. But Warwick asked me to interview in January 1970, when I was still 16. I had to go for an interview in Coventry, and I took my mum with me. The interview was a total humiliation. Obviously I had my injections and sandwiches with me, so I was well prepared. But the Dean of the university was otherwise engaged, and so the Head Student interviewed me. He obviously didn't like the look of the 16-year-old nerd sitting before him, and the interview went extremely badly. For instance, with regard to conveyancing, he asked me the question, "What do you need to build a house?"

Nowadays, I understand he meant things like planning permission. But the 16-year-old me said, "I think a big pile of bricks would be a start. And some bags of cement."

"Hmm," he said. "That's not quite the answer I was looking for."

At the end of the interview, I asked him, "When will I hear?" He said, "Very soon." I think, in those pre-electronic days, it was the first time a rejection beat the train back to Liverpool.

So that didn't get my higher education off to a good start, although I wasn't very keen on going to Warwick University. I had always had my sights set on Liverpool, which was widely considered the best law school outside Oxbridge, mostly because the Dean was Professor David Seaborne Davies, the brains behind the Theft Act 1968. But that wasn't the only reason.

On April Fool's Day, the day before my 17th birthday, I received the greatest present I could imagine. I witnessed my beloved boys in blue being crowned champions of England. How could I move away and miss watching an Everton side which included the Holy Trinity of Howard Kendall, Alan Ball, and Colin Harvey?

And another consideration was gastronomic. Mum's cooking was fantastic on a Friday night for our Sabbath meal, the highlight of which was good old fashioned Jewish chicken soup, often described as kosher penicillin, and tasty roast chicken and roast potatoes. How could I move away from that? But perhaps there was another, more pressing, reason to stay…

I was in the foyer at Liverpool University when my dear friend Richard Isaacson spotted me. Richard was my barrister many years later when I represented Jon Venables in the James Bulger case. He was gloriously flamboyant, the life and soul of any party, and like another older brother to me. He was head of the debating society, born to be a QC, and in his second year at the time. He bustled over to me and exclaimed, "Hello, Little Lolly!" - he always called me Little Lolly - "Come for your interview, have you?"

I said, "Yes, I've come to see Professor Seaborne Davies." I was mildly wetting myself at the prospect.

"Oh, you'll be fine!" Richard said.

"What do I say to him?" I asked, nervously.

"Oh," he said, "just prostrate yourself before him!" And he

demonstrated with a flourish.

Richard died suddenly in 1998 of a heart attack. In a tribute in The Lawyer, Judge David Clarke QC said Richard was "in command of all the weapons available to an advocate - the rapier, the bludgeon, and the steam roller when it was called for." If anything, that understated the great Richard Isaacson QC.

In any case, I decided against prostrating myself in front of the man behind the Theft Act 1968, mostly because I didn't want to get myself arrested. Instead, I sat through the interview sensibly. Prof. Seaborne Davies noted my age, and he said, "Why don't you stay down for another year? You're only 17."

The last thing I wanted to do was repeat another year. I told him, "I do not want to go back to school. I want to come here." So he put me on the waiting list, with grades of A, B, and C to be assured of my place at Liverpool. And so, every morning, before my revision marathon, I would play the record that would inspire me to success, namely *ABC,* by the Jackson 5. It didn't quite work out for me. Instead of ABC, I managed to achieve CBC, not quite a Number One hit, but enough to get me into Liverpool. I thought, "Wow, that's great. But how am I going to cope with diabetes?"

That was it, the real reason I had to stay. I often ask myself if, in hindsight, I would have grown up quicker had I chosen to leave home. I have to admit I didn't have the confidence to live away from home as a newly diagnosed diabetic, despite the giant strides I'd achieved. That would have to change. And my friend Uli would have a lot to do with that…

4
Reprieve From A Death Sentence

When I was in hospital for the first time, under the care of Dr Heinz Fuld, I decided I needed to get to the bottom of what caused diabetes and any other information I could get my hands on. That's how I discovered the work of Frederick Banting, Charles Best, and their associates.

There's much less ignorance about diabetes these days, partly because it seems much more prevalent, particularly the Type 2 variant, which is associated with greater obesity.

Diabetes itself was first chronicled as long ago as the Egyptian era. They noticed that flies would gather around the urine of a diabetic, because of its high sugar content, and the Egyptians gave it the appropriate, if hardly flattering, nickname of "peeing disease".

Why do diabetics have high sugar content in their urine, you might ask? Well, when a normal, non-diabetic person eats, their body breaks down carbohydrates in food and drink into glucose, the sort of sugar you get in Lucozade. This glucose goes straight into the blood stream.

And in a normal person, the pancreas produces insulin, which is a hormone crucial in breaking down sugars into energy - it acts like a carburettor in a car. Insulin is created by beta cells, which are within a part of the pancreas called the islets of Langerhans

Type 1 diabetes - which I have - is an autoimmune disease which attacks these beta cells in the pancreas. Fewer beta cells means less insulin, and, without a healthy supply of insulin the sugar levels rise to the extent that excess sugar flows into the urine.

In time, high blood sugar levels can damage your eyes, heart, feet and kidneys. In fact, the effect on the kidneys is often what causes diabetes to be diagnosed. The kidneys are a filtration system, and attempt to get rid of the excess glucose. This can cause the sufferer to urinate a lot. It can also make the sufferer extremely thirsty.

That was what tipped off my dad that I might be diabetic, and the high sugar levels in my blood and urine confirmed it.

Diabetes was in effect a terminal illness before 1921. That was the year that two more of my heroes, Frederick Banting and Charles Best, of the University of Toronto, isolated insulin. The term "insulin" had already been coined by an English physiologist called Edward Sharpey-Schafer, the man who discovered adrenaline. Sharpey-Schafer had theorised that a substance from the pancreas was responsible for diabetes, and Banting thought he could find a way of extracting insulin from a dog's pancreas without the enzymes in the pancreas destroying it.

He discussed his ideas with John McLeod, Professor of Physiology at Toronto, who provided him with experimental facilities and lent him one of his best students, Charles Best. Banting and Best, along with biochemist James Collip, set about their work. On 30 July 1921, a diabetic dog was injected with insulin and its blood glucose levels returned to normal.

The researchers then discovered that they could extract insulin from cattle and pigs. It was time to try their discovery on humans.

And so, on 11 January 1922, the first human insulin trial took place - 14-year-old Canadian Leonard Thompson at Toronto General Hospital. Leonard had been drifting in and out of a diabetic coma, and weighed only 65 pounds, and could hardly lift his head from his pillow. His father, in desperation, agreed to allow his son to have the first-ever insulin injection. Leonard failed to improve after his first injection of crude canine insulin, but the researchers refused to give up, attributing their failure to an allergic reaction. Collip was tasked with refining the insulin for human consumption. The second injection, with a purer solution, immediately took

Leonard's blood sugar levels back to normal, and his symptoms disappeared.

The work of the researchers earned a Nobel Prize for Medicine in 1923, but it caused acrimony among the team for the rest of their lives. The prize was awarded to Banting and McLeod, and Banting was furious, believing that the professor was taking too much credit for his and Best's discovery. He shared his Nobel prize money with Best, while McLeod shared his prize money with Collip. It was only in later years that the contribution of all four men was appreciated.

Soon after Leonard Thompson's successful treatment, the medical firm Eli Lilly started large-scale production of insulin, but the patent remained with the British Medical Research Council, to prevent profiteering. In the years following, manufacturers developed a variety of slower-acting insulins.

Insulin from cattle and pigs was used for many years to treat diabetes and saved millions of lives, but it wasn't perfect, as I can testify. I felt as if I were in second gear for years. It was only when I moved on to "human" insulin that I felt properly in tune. This synthetic "human" insulin was created in 1978 using genetically engineered E. coli bacteria to produce the insulin. Eli Lilly went on in 1982 to sell the first commercial biosynthetic human insulin, named Humulin. But it would be years after that before I would give it a go.

While Leonard Thompson made a full recovery, and had much improved health, he died 13 years after his first insulin injection of pneumonia, related to his diabetes. But the year after Leonard's injection, another young boy received his first insulin treatment, and his story was much happier.

In 1921, seven-year-old Alan Nabarro was diagnosed with Type 1 diabetes. It was a death sentence. Or it would have been had it not been for his uncle David, who was a doctor at Great Ormond Street Hospital. He had heard of the groundbreaking work being done by Banting and Best in Ontario, and he bombarded the Canadian researchers with telegrams begging them for insulin. Frustratingly for David Nabarro and his family, he was told that insulin was not yet available for distribution. Alan's family were then placed in touch with a consultant in Brussels, a Dr Devos, who put Alan on a near-starvation diet, with a fast of spinach and cream once a week. This unchanging diet kept the little boy alive until 1923 when he was finally allowed to have his first insulin injection.

I see a lot of myself in Alan. Like me, he took control of his own condition from an early age. Like me, he produced little diet sheets which told him what he could eat every day, including a special Bar Mitzvah sheet. He qualified as a solicitor too. And he experienced ridicule because he took injections in public toilets. His letters, which are available from the Royal College of Physicians archives, tell of a frightening incident, when he was 11, of being verbally abused by a stranger in a restaurant toilet while he was injecting himself with insulin. I suffered similar ridicule when I weighed my food in public view in cafés and restaurants. Alan told his consultant, Geoffrey Harrison, about the incident, and Dr Harrison drew up a certificate for Alan to carry with him at all times, explaining his condition and the need for insulin injections.

When he became an adult, he joined the British Diabetic Association - now known as Diabetes UK - and spent the rest of his life travelling the world promoting diabetes awareness. He died on 22 March 1977, one of the longest living people with diabetes at that time, and the British Diabetic Association decided to honour his memory with the Alan Nabarro Medal, which is awarded to people who have lived with diabetes for 50 years. I cannot tell you how proud I felt when I was awarded this beautiful medal in 2018.

If this book has just a fraction of the impact of the life of Alan Nabarro in spreading the word about diabetes and how to live with it, I'll be a happy man.

Today, diabetes is no longer a death sentence. People with Type 1 diabetes are at the top of every profession. In the fields of showbiz and sport, the likes of Pakistani cricketer Wasim Akram, Oscar-winning actress Halle Berry, boxer Buster Douglas, comedian Ed Gamble, footballer Gary Mabbutt, rock singer Bret Michaels, actor James Norton, and singer Vanessa Williams have Type 1 diabetes. In politics, the US Supreme Court judge Sonia Sotomayor and the former British Prime Minister Theresa May have risen to the peak of their field while managing their Type 1 diabetes. Most of them are alive today because of the work that Banting, Best, McLeod, and Collip did 100 years ago. And so am I, more than half a century after my diagnosis.

5
Over The Berlin Wall

Professor Seaborne Davies was right that I was too young to start university at 17. I started at Liverpool in October 1970 and, frankly, I felt completely awful immediately. I wasn't well enough to go to Freshers' Week, and I only went to one party in my first year. The step-up from school to university would have been bad enough for a normal 17-year-old, but I was a young 17-year-old, more like a 15-year-old. And I was a 17-year-old with recently diagnosed diabetes, which I was only just starting to manage.

The good professor had lived quite the life before I encountered him. For a start, he was one of the shortest-lived MPs of the 20th century. When David Lloyd George was elevated to the Lords after five decades as MP for Caernarvon Boroughs, David Seaborne Davies was adopted by the Liberal Party as his successor candidate. He beat Plaid Cymru in the by-election forced by Lloyd George's resignation in the dying days of World War II. But there was a swift General Election following the war, and he was booted out by the Conservatives. Soon after, he arrived at Liverpool, where he was appointed to the Chair of Common Law at the university's law faculty. And in 1968, as a member of the Criminal Law Revision Committee, he was instrumental in the writing of the Theft Act of that year. As far as criminal law went, he was something of a rock star.

Professor Seaborne Davies gave me a piece of advice that I have never forgotten. He was my lecturer for criminal law in the first year, and I was finding criminal law pretty tough. It wasn't so much that the course was beyond me. It was that I was ill and lacking in energy. I remember trudging up the stairs feeling terrible, and jealously looking at my classmates going to parties and going out for pints and living that student life, and I was going home on the 86 bus to my mum and dad. The Christmas exams came around, and the pass mark in Liverpool was 33%. You would imagine that you'd just have to get your name right, and you'd be well on the way to a pass mark.

Not for me. I got my Christmas exam back and Seaborne Davies had marked it as 30%, with 33% in brackets after it. And on the paper he had written, "I have given you a pass mark, but may I strongly recommend that you do not take up criminal law as your profession?"

Doubtless there are some clients who would applaud that advice, and wish I had taken it. But I was determined to prove him wrong. I had decided that I did not want to go to the Bar. I wanted to be a solicitor. Years before, at Sunday lunch, the front door bell went at the surgery in Storrsdale Road. A man had come off his motorbike and he was covered in blood. And we had to interrupt our roast beef for my dad to stitch him up in the surgery. He was in a terrible mess, and that's when I decided that I didn't want to be a doctor. I couldn't stand the sight of blood. No, I'd rather be a criminal lawyer and represent the bloke who knocked him off his bike…

By Easter term, I'd gone up to 50%. I never got much beyond that. Even now, I probably know more criminal law than I think, but, as the late great Frank Carson used to say, "It's the way you tell 'em." I was never an academic, but many of the guys sitting next to me in university were academics, and I felt inadequate in comparison. There was David Aubrey, who was very bright, and who became a top judge in Liverpool. Brian Leveson, the Rt Hon Lord Justice Leveson, who led the inquiry into conduct of the press following the News of the World's phone-hacking scandal, was in the year above me. He'd been at Liverpool College too. He was the best friend of Richard Isaacson, who had told me to prostrate myself before Seaborne Davies at my interview. You could tell Brian was destined for greatness at an early age. He and Richard had been to a Jewish summer school somewhere in the south of England when they were about 13. When it became time for them to buy souvenirs for their parents, Richard bought some sticks of rock, the sort of thing one would imagine a 13-year-old boy would bring back from the seaside. Brian, on the other hand, bought a set of sherry schooners. Richard said, "Why the hell are you buying your parents sherry schooners?"

Brian replied, "It's about time they improved their social circle." Now that's what it takes to become a top judge.

Another classmate, who became a very prominent accident lawyer, was Michael Pickavance. On his first day - when everybody else was in jeans and T-shirts - he rolled up at his first lecture in a green, tweed, three-piece suit. He was terribly posh and far back. And every five minutes his hand would shoot up and he'd say, "Excuse meeee!" Question after question after question. We had a reunion a few years ago and all of my classmates had done so well. I was proud of my year. I was the only flop, really. Though you're reading my book and not theirs, so we all know who's the real winner here...

I didn't feel like a winner at the time, though. My life at university in that first year was low-grade, partly because I was at home. But also I didn't have a lot of energy in those days. I wasn't permanently ill, but I wasn't right. I was dragging. And then the stress of exams became too much. It caused my blood sugar to escalate, and I had great difficulty sleeping. At the end of the first year we were studying Roman law and I learnt the syllabus off by heart. But following the end of the exam I couldn't get it out of my head. I was in a bad way. And so, in May 1971, back into my life came Dr Heinz Fuld.

I needed a rest, and I needed my daily insulin dosage to be adjusted, so Dr Fuld had me admitted to Sefton General Hospital again, and I was kept in for about a week. My immediate instinct was to take advantage of the situation and have a rest after such a testing year. Sadly for me, our Teutonic disciplinarian had other ideas.

He found me one day lying on my bed reading.

"What are you doing?" he asked, pointedly.

"I'm resting, Doctor Fuld," I replied - not the best retort to an athletic god like Heinz Fuld.

His reaction was merciless.

"I want you to run around the building all day. No wonder you support Everton - they are so lazy. You should support Liverpool [heaven forbid]. We are so workmanlike!"

He shook me out of my lethargy and I was back home a week later. I wouldn't be here without him because he was so strict. Yes, he was a taskmaster, but he made me fit. Even though he was a bloody nuisance and I was freezing cold and wanted to stay in and read, he had me training. He was my physical and psychological mentor. I love him for it in retrospect. At the time I hated him.

I was a lot better after that and my second and third years were to be a great improvement. I passed them, because then I was 18 or 19 and reaching the age that I should have been when I started university.

So I had started to take control of my diabetes. Sadly, my grandpa's own strict regime was not infallible, and my nerdish knowledge of diabetes came to prove to be life-saving when, in 1971, my grandmother telephoned to say Sidney was having an afternoon snooze and she couldn't wake him up for his 6pm supper.

I suspected something was amiss and ran round the corner to their house. It was immediately clear to me that grandpa was having a deep hypoglycaemic episode which had gone past the stage of taking a bite of a Mars bar. He was unconscious and grandma was in a right state. I told her that prayer was not the answer on this occasion and I rushed to my dad's surgery and dragged out his partner, Dr John Newman - a nice chap, but as dull as a Tuesday in February. He was an eternal bachelor, who may have been academically sound, but he was no James Bond when it came to charisma and charm. I was told that on a very rare date he bought a young lady a gin and tonic, but ruined it all by telling her to drink it more slowly because it cost a fortune.

I made it quite clear that unless we got glucose into Sidney in the next few minutes he could die. I eventually bullied and persuaded Dr Newman to follow me round to their house with a glucose phial and a syringe. Within minutes, Sidney had an intravenous injection of pure glucose, and in no time he came round and was as close to being right as rain as he ever could be.

I was very grateful to my dad's partner and, indeed, I was proud of myself for, quite frankly, saving grandpa Sidney's life.

I was a little concerned that I hadn't done the right thing so I telephoned my Germanic hero Heinz Fuld and told him what I'd done. I still remember his comment…

"Laurence, you deserve an honorary MD."

A couple of years later, in 1973, Dr Fuld, who had kept in touch with me to make sure I was still exercising, called to invite me to a football match. His beloved and workmanlike Liverpool were playing Dynamo Dresden from his homeland in the UEFA Cup, and he wanted me to join him in the director's box at Anfield - a thought that filled me, a devoted Evertonian, with horror.

At about 9pm, when the match still had more than 20 minutes to go, he announced that he was giving a talk at the nearby Newsham General Hospital and that we must leave now. That wasn't a problem for me… but once we were outside he told me that we were behind his Germanic schedule and, in his words, we must trot a little bit. Trot?! Remember, he was in his 70s and I was 21. He shot off like an Olympic sprinter, leaving me gasping in his wake. I feared that if I didn't keep up with him I'd be sentenced to another spell in Sefton General for intensive physical training.

I eventually caught up with him. He said nothing, but the look on his face clearly expressed his disappointment in my lack of athleticism.

The year 1973 would be one of the most significant in my life. I took my final exams. But, just a week before them, my beloved grandpa Sidney died, which was awful timing. Even worse than its impact on my exams, his death made me miss an Everton home match against Wolves. We beat them 2-1, so I forgave him...

Following university, my next target was to qualify as a solicitor. The mountain I faced was steeper than any university degree, in the form of a six-month course in Chester, starting in August with solicitors finals in February. But in the weeks before my graduation ceremony, I found myself at a loose end. I'd finished my university studies, and now I wanted to stretch myself in a different way. I wanted an adventure.

In 1973, going to Berlin really was an adventure. It was the height of the Cold War, and the Wall split the city down the middle, the free world in the west and Soviet-style communism in the east. And, of course, as somebody managing diabetes, I had to take my insulin with me and to make sure I had food. I've been carrying Mars Bars or Crunchie bars with me since 1968. And I think if you were to look in some of my old pockets, you'll find that the sell-by date is probably about 1972. My chocolate bars fester in my pocket for ages. There's probably an Aztec in there somewhere. I also had a few packs of chewing gum, which I took everywhere at the time.

I flew off to Berlin and landed at the very airport where Hitler landed, a thought which gave me chills. And I was greeted at the airport by my old friend Uli, who picked me up and took me to his apartment. Uli was the reason I chose Berlin. It was great to be reunited with "my other big brother", but I think it gave me some reassurance to know that I wasn't entirely on my own for this big adventure. Uli lived near Walther Schreiber Platz underground station. There was a disco nearby called The 45, which, presumably, referred to the RPM of a record single, rather than VE Day...

Uli shared his apartment, with a perpetual student called Ahmed, who came from Alexandria in Egypt. He was in one room. I was in another. And Uli was in the third.

In those days, I wore my Star of David. I wasn't at all religious - those long services at Greenbank Road synagogue had put paid to that notion - but I was loyal to Judaism and Zionism, and Ahmed was equally loyal to Islam. And, as is usual in history, Egypt and Israel were not exactly bosom buddies at the time. Nevertheless, Ahmed - who looked a bit like Mohamed Salah, so, in retrospect, I'm surprised by this – and I got on extremely well. He was very friendly and he spoke broken English.

However, I noticed, when I went to bed the first night, left on my bed was an English translation of a speech that President Nasser made to the Egyptian nation, basically condemning Israel to hell. I wasn't taking that. I thought, "Right, revenge is sweet," and so the next night I took off my Star of David and draped it over his pillow. All I could hear was terrible Egyptian screams coming from next door. We decided to have a truce after that.

At this point, Uli's mum took ill in Munich and I was left alone with Ahmed in the flat. We both survived it. But we used to get the bus to University every day, and at the bus stop one day, Ahmed said, "I'd like you to meet some friends of mine". So I thought, "Oh, hello there. That's nice." So I met this friend of Ahmed and he introduced me to some other friends. He said, "These are my friends from Jerusalem."

I thought, "Oh, good, one of the boys!"

And he said, "This is Abdul from East Jerusalem."

"Ah, hello, Abdul," I said, and then he introduced me to Anwar from Damascus. These guys were lovely, because when people from different backgrounds talk to each other, they usually are. Anwar even said, "If ever you're in Damascus, please drop in." I must say that if Middle East peace talks were down to the four of us, thousands of lives could have been saved and bloodshed would have been a thing of the past. We all got on very well and spent a very happy week together.

It was while I was in Berlin that I suffered my only instance of anti-Semitism so far. Two days after I met my new Middle Eastern pals, it was the Fourth of July. The university was next to the US Army base. Students then, as now, were usually lefties and didn't particularly like Americans, and there was a demonstration. I wanted to watch the demonstration, because what was the point of being in Berlin otherwise? But I didn't want to take part in it because I actually loved America. Tempers flared, and the West German police charged in, chucking tear gas. So the students retreated and Laurence Lee, almost LLB, was caught offside, as I often was in the football pitch. Strangely, tear gas can't tell the difference between an anti-American protester, and a pro-American observer. I can still feel the pain in my eyes today.

Lesson learned, I managed to find my way, as if I had a white stick, back to the university campus, and miraculously I didn't get arrested. That night Uli returned from his mother's and he said, "Look, for goodness' sake, would you just stay out of trouble? Tomorrow, it's the Fifth of July. There are lovely botanical gardens in Berlin. It's baking. Would you please go to the cafe there, take a book, and chill out?"

So I took Uli's advice, and went to the cafe. It was the height of summer, and extremely hot. I was reading my book and a friendly German waiter came over to me. We started talking. I was speaking German, talking about football, and thoroughly enjoying myself. Everything was perfect. And, as it got hotter, I took my sweater off, and started undoing my shirt and he kept coming back, plying me with coffee and tea, and just generally looking after me. Then, when my shirt was unbuttoned, my Star of David was revealed... it was if he had switched off completely. He stared at it and then he shouted at the top of his voice, *"Geschlossen"* - closed - "We are shut! Get out!"

So I stumbled out, shocked. And then I started laughing to myself because on my tab were four coffees and three cups of tea, and I hadn't yet paid. So, anti-Semitism nil, Laurence Lee FC one.

A couple of days later, Uli, who at that point was a teacher in Berlin, decided that we were going to East Berlin the next day.

When I was planning my trip, I had been to travel agents in Liverpool telling them I intended to visit the east of the city, and they said, "You can't go, that's impossible. How can an English person go to East Berlin?" I explained this to Uli, but he said, "Rubbish, you're going."

"How are we going to work this out?" I asked.

"Leave it with me," he said.

So the next day, we met up at Friedrichstrasse, which was the border. Weirdly, Friedrichstrasse at ground level and above was West Berlin. But Friedrichstrasse underground was East Berlin. So it was a three-dimensional border. When we got there, we were split into three groups: West Berliners, West Germans, and foreigners, or Auslander, which meant me. Uli and his class split into two, because half of them were from West Germany, as was Uli, and the other half hailed from West Berlin. The West Germans and West Berliners got through the border pretty quickly. I, on the other hand, was led into a dungeon, was given a piece of paper with a number on, as if I were waiting for a shoe fitting in the children's section of Clarks, exchanged West German currency to the East German sort, and waited for my number to be called out. During the process, I was searched several times. When eventually I was let out, I was shown to a door that was similar to the fire exit from an old-fashioned cinema. I pushed the bar to exit, and came out into a grotty alleyway. This passage took me back to the main unterdenlinden, which was the border area, and Uli and his class said, "God, where the hell have you been?"

I said, "Don't ask, just don't ask."

When we got out onto the main thoroughfare, all we could see were tanks going backwards and forwards, and posters stating "Socialism is best". We sat on the banks of the river Spree before going to the place that was the purpose of our trip. The plan was that we would go to the Goethe theatre to watch - God, how could I even tolerate five minutes of it? - *Coriolanus* translated from Shakespearean English to German by Schiller. And we went into this grand

61

theatre that Hitler used to frequent. It was an incredible building, but it was warm, and within 10 minutes, I was asleep and the students were dozing off. And after a while, Uli, who was a very cool dude, basically said, "Look, sod this for a game of soldiers, guys. You've got a choice, you can either stay here and watch the rest of this crap, or come back to my flat for a party." So you can guess what the poll said…

So in no time we were in a department store, because there were no private restaurants in East Berlin. We went into the equivalent of George Henry Lee's or John Lewis. Well there weren't any John Lewis department stores in East Berlin. It was more like TJ Hughes. And I ordered chicken and chips. As Ken Dodd might have said, "There was more meat on a budgie's chest", and, believe me, I'd have rather had the budgie. It was just awful. I don't know how people survived over there.

So then we decided to go back to Checkpoint Charlie and get back to the West and I was questioned by this young East German guard, a beautiful, if glacial, lady, of around 23. She was *Nikita,* from the Elton John video, a tough East German guard. She was distinctly unimpressed by my insulin and didn't appear to know what it was. And I also had some chewing gum on me in silver foil. I have to admit that if you were an East German border guard who knew very little about diabetes, and you were confronted by a 20-year-old, long-haired lout of a foreign westerner carrying needles, a phial of drugs, and some silver foil, you would probably be suspicious too.

She asked me if I had any medical evidence to prove I was diabetic. I was beginning to get a bit panicky. And then she demanded, "And where did you buy this chewing gum?"

I stammered, "I bought it at Barrington's in Greenhill Road!" I was fairly sure, even at the time, that she was unlikely to be familiar with Barrington's in Greenhill Road, but you never know. Anyway, eventually, I think, just to get rid of me, she said, "Oh, go back to the West, for God's sake." And when I got back to the West, I literally put my hand on the ground and kissed it. And we went back to Uli's flat and I just got bladdered on low-sugar lager.

So that was my trip to Berlin. It was a great trip. But more than that, it gave me the biggest boost because that was my first trip abroad on my own. There were no hurdles I couldn't leap after that.

When I returned, I graduated, and started my six-month solicitor course at Chester, which was very hard. I was still living at home at the time, along with Michael. And we started our articles at around the same time. Doing your articles is best described as an apprenticeship for solicitors, in which you work at a firm. And I was taken on by Cyril Carr.

Cyril Carr was a councillor for the Liberal Party in Liverpool. I started with him in February 1974, just in time for the first general election of that year. Cyril was campaigning for the Liberals in Garston constituency against Eddie Loyden for Labour. And my first two weeks of articles were spent up a ladder campaigning for the Liberals. Cyril said to me, at the start of my articles, "You're going up in the world." I didn't realise he was so literal.

Cyril's dad was my grandfather Sidney's best friend. I'd tried articles with one of my dad's patients, at a small suburban firm in Garston. But Cyril indicated, because of friendship with my parents, that he had a place for me. He didn't actually have a place at all, because his office was packed. There were two other article clerks already, called Stan and Rod. I was very junior to them. There were two qualified solicitors. And there was no way I was ever going to survive in there, I thought. But gradually, as the years went by, two emigrated, one went to another firm, the lady solicitor became pregnant, and there was only me by the end. So, by the time I qualified, there was only one other solicitor, Rod, who, even though he was more experienced than me, was not Cyril's blue-eyed boy. That honour fell to me. I was very go-ahead at the time, and Cyril would often defer to me. Although Cyril did once say to me, "If I'd known you were an Evertonian, I'd never have taken you on," because he was a staunch Red. It was a Red firm, but I thought, "I'm going to change all that." After he died, I took over the firm. It's now a bastion of blue and white - all the signage is blue and white - and all the staff… Well, they don't have to be blue and white because I'd be in breach of employment law, but they know any expression of being a Red is forbidden.

Cyril's office was at 28 Exchange Street East opposite the Town Hall. So every day, after work, I would come out of the bulilding, turn left, walk down to Dale Street, cross the road, and end up at Gerald Strong's, in the State Building, where my brother Michael was articled. Michael was a very naughty boy. He pretended to support Liverpool, just to wind me up, and he succeeded. He would tease me before the match. He'd say, "Are you going to Goodison today?"

And I'd say, "Yes, I am."

He'd say, "I'll make you a bet. I bet I'll score more than Everton do." And of course he did. He'd be off to meet his lady friends. Michael was very handsome and dashing. He used to go mad because people said he looked like Elliott Gould. He hated Elliott Gould for daring to impersonate him.

Michael and I were neck-and-neck with articles. He didn't go to uni, but he was at the Polytechnic, and they had a well-respected law school run by John and Mary Conkerton, a married couple, who were patients of my dad. They both died in 1979, but every few years since then the Conkerton Memorial Lecture has been organised by Liverpool Law Society. They were brilliant lawyers and lecturers, and, in fact, Mr Conkerton taught me Accounts Law. He was really good. And Michael would have sailed through his exams had it not been for, well, outside distractions… He was articled with Gerald Strong, who was a formidable character. Gerald himself was a gruff, round-shaped, little man. He was the total opposite of Cyril, because Cyril was very meek and mild. He was like Corporal Wilson in *Dad's Army,* whereas Gerald was Captain Mainwaring, both in shape and behaviour.

For example, Wilson - Cyril Carr - would say, "Oh, it's a quarter to five, Laurence. You might as well go. Have a nice evening."

As Michael and I travelled to work together, I'd have to go to Gerald Strong's office to wait for my brother. Gerald would bark at me, "What time do you call this?"

"Five o' clock, Mr Strong."

"Five o'clock?! The day's only just begun!"

He and Michael would shout at each other. I wouldn't have dared speak like that to Cyril. I wouldn't have any reason to, because Cyril and I would never argue, except about football.

But Gerald and Michael would argue fiercely about minor things, like whether "we should" or "we would" would be at the start of a letter - "We should be grateful…" or "We would be grateful…" - and my brother would call him an old bugger.

"Don't you talk to me like that!" Gerald would say.

And Michael would say, "Oh, I'm going home. I've had enough of you today, Gerald."

And Gerald would cheerfully say, "OK, Mike, see you tomorrow." And it would all be forgotten by the next morning.

Michael always stood up for himself. He was a real feisty, bossy guy. He had a flat of his own… for other purposes. It was, shall we say, a social pied-à-terre?

But he lived at home. It was a happy, eventful household. My poor mum was beaten into submission by three males. My dad was a real Yorkshireman. He used to call her "Mother". And on Friday nights we had our Sabbath dinner, and, much as I loved my mum's Friday night dinners, she was no Nigella Lawson. Her chicken soup tasted lovely, but unfortunately, she couldn't get the temperature right, and he'd shout, "Mother, this bloody soup's cold."

"I'm sorry about that, David," she'd say. So she'd take it away and reheat it and he'd burn his mouth on this later. And he'd say, "It's either too bloody hot or too bloody cold."

But she was a good Jewish mama, and absolutely all-encompassing. Everything would wash over her head. And no matter who shouted at her, she'd say, "Oooh! Never mind, dear." She was absolutely amazing. She'd just go into the other room and start writing more poetry. She wrote one when she was 15 called Sleep, which the Radio Merseyside presenter Roger Phillips used to love hearing, because it was very therapeutic. You would feel absolutely relaxed when you read it. I used to joke with her, "You were only 15 when you wrote this?! You must have had a spliff before you wrote it."

"How dare you?!" she would say. "A spliff?! I never touched drugs!" Poor woman.

I'd often see Michael at the Mercantile Cafe. This was a subterranean restaurant on Castle Street, on the site currently occupied by Olive, and all the businessmen went there. At the Mercantile, the food was great, but you'd pay on trust, just like in Anderson's on Exchange Street East. You'd have a tray and you'd pick various things, as in a cafeteria. There was a very formidable lady on the till and you'd go up to her with your scotch egg and sausages, or whatever you had chosen that day, and say, "One and six!" But really it should have been three shillings and sixpence. So they went bankrupt, basically. They never learnt that you can't trust lawyers.

I carried on with my articles after Cyril had lost the election and I soon realised that conveyancing was not for me. There was nothing I liked about it. But, towards the end of the period, I said to Cyril, "Look, let's turn to crime." Cyril didn't know anything about criminal law, but I was very persuasive in those days, and I said, "Look, you'll make more money out of criminal law." Oh, how times have changed! Also, because Cyril was on the city council, he was a good advocate. So we went onto the duty solicitors' rota, and every time we were on duty we'd pick up around 10 new cases, which was good for the firm. And it was good for me too, because every time we were duty solicitor we went for a meal in Chinatown afterwards. And when we went in he'd always say, "Before you do anything, wash your hands. Dirty defendants!" And some of them were very grubby. But we built up a small criminal practice and things were starting to look good for me and Michael. Nothing could have prepared me for what was about to happen.

On the night of December 21 1975, I had gone to the Brook-house pub on Smithdown Road with my soon-to-be first wife. It was a Sunday evening and I had what I can only describe as a pre-monition as I was about to pay the bill. I started getting these terrible stomach cramps, like a knife in my gut, to the extent that I just left money on the table, didn't wait for change, and came out and slumped over my car. I went home and Michael was there and he said to me, "Don't worry, Lol, you'll be all right." That was the last time I saw him.

I will never forget the anguished screams of my poor mother the next morning, when she found his lifeless body in bed.

His death remains inexplicable to me. One day he was the Michael I always knew, the next he was gone, and we'll never know why. The only closure I had was that the Merseyside County Coroner, Roy Barter, recorded an open verdict.

The funeral was on December 23, in accordance with Jewish tradition, and then we were whisked off to Leeds. I took my books with me, because I studying for my finals, which were only six weeks away. Greenbank Drive Synagogue was so understanding. We were meant to have seven nights of prayer, but the synagogue told us, "You can have just one night, then go to Leeds. Get out of here." And we needed to, because it was such a unique, horrible situation. I still remember the thud of the soil on the grave, and that sound is haunting. He was buried at the Jewish cemetery on Long Lane, next to my mum and dad now. It was just a nightmare, and so awful to see all his friends in tears. And I thought, "How am I going to get over this?"

Even now, every time I walk past Gerald Strong's office on Dale Street — and that office is long gone, replaced first by the State nightclub, and now by a gymnasium — I inwardly shed a tear and wonder what life might have been like had Michael lived. I think we'd have killed each other, if we'd worked together, because we were so different in those days. I was very shy.

But as soon as he died, I took over his boisterousness, his lack of shyness, because I had to support my mum and dad. And I took over the outspoken gregariousness of Michael. It was almost like a transformation, as if it was implanted in me from him.

I only ever saw him once in court, but my brother Michael was cool, even in the way he dressed for court. He wouldn't wear the old-fashioned black suit, he'd have a blazer, smart tie, and trousers. And he looked so damn smart in them. Nobody ever complained. Everybody respected him. He fought his corner.

Michael's death put me off track for my final solicitors exams, which were due in February 1976, but I buried myself in my books, and passed the remaining exams in time for my articles to end. I qualified in June 1976, and went down to the Law Society in London to receive my award from the Lord Chancellor, Lord El-wyn-Jones. Cyril told me, "You're going to be asked by the Lord Chancellor about what it means to be a solicitor. Somehow get the word 'integrity' into it."

So I ended up on stage, about to get my award for qualifying after a horrendous solicitors finals course in Chester, and the Lord Chancellor said to me, "And what do you think are the main qualities to be a solicitor?"

"Oh, integrity, sir," I said. I could see his eyes rolling. I must have been the 95th qualified solicitor to say that. There was obviously somebody outside selling tips on what to say. Nice one, Cyril.

The day I qualified in June 1976, Cyril buzzed down and said, "Congratulations! Monday morning, you're on your own. You'll never get me into that bloody court again." And on that Monday morning, I went to St Helens Magistrates' for my first case, and I forgot to apply for Legal Aid until after the case. And I asked the clerk, who was like Basil Fawlty, "Can I have Legal Aid, please?" And he said, "No! You're too late." So I had to go back to Cyril and tell him we'd just done a charity case. It didn't go down too well, and I never made that mistake again.

From then on, I was in court every day, and I have been ever since.

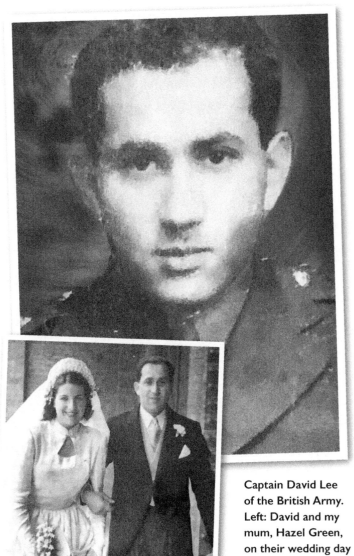

Captain David Lee of the British Army. Left: David and my mum, Hazel Green, on their wedding day at Greenbank Drive Synagogue on 18 June 1947

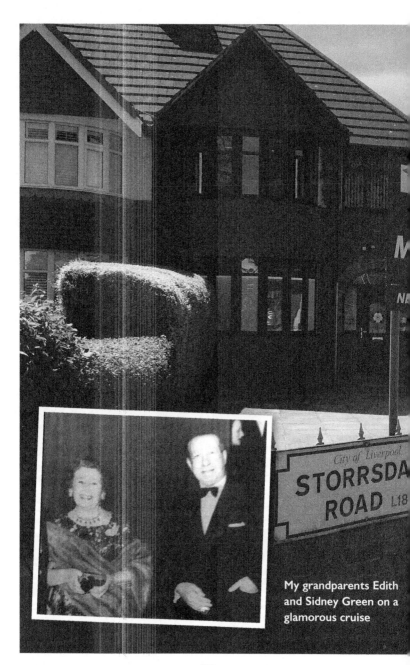

City of Liverpool
STORRSDA
ROAD L18

My grandparents Edith and Sidney Green on a glamorous cruise

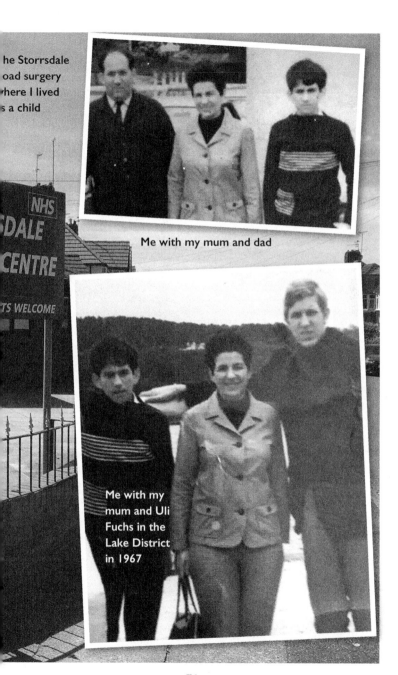

he Storrsdale
oad surgery
here I lived
s a child

NHS
SDALE
CENTRE
TS WELCOME

Me with my mum and dad

Me with my
mum and Uli
Fuchs in the
Lake District
in 1967

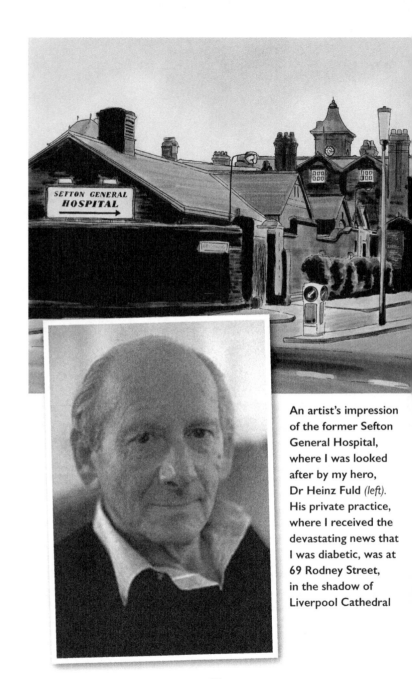

An artist's impression of the former Sefton General Hospital, where I was looked after by my hero, Dr Heinz Fuld *(left)*. His private practice, where I received the devastating news that I was diabetic, was at 69 Rodney Street, in the shadow of Liverpool Cathedral

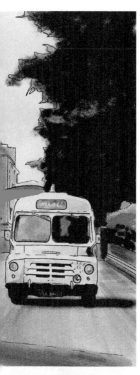

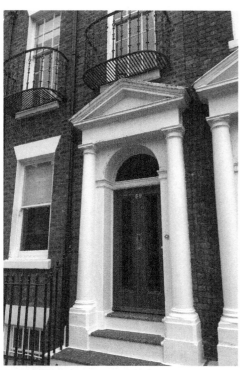

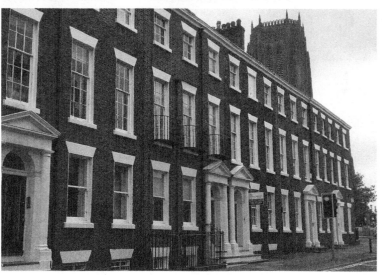

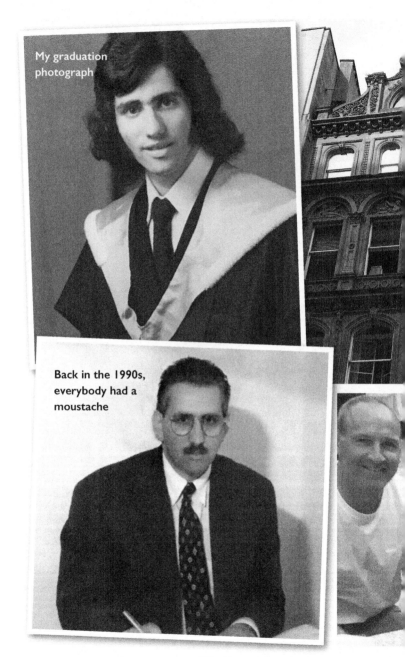

My graduation photograph

Back in the 1990s, everybody had a moustache

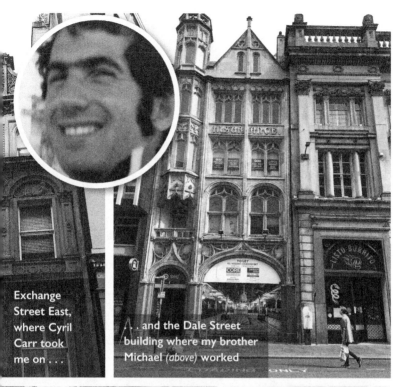

Exchange Street East, where Cyril Carr took me on . . .

. . . and the Dale Street building where my brother Michael *(above)* worked

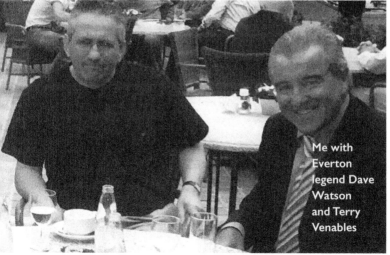

Me with Everton legend Dave Watson and Terry Venables

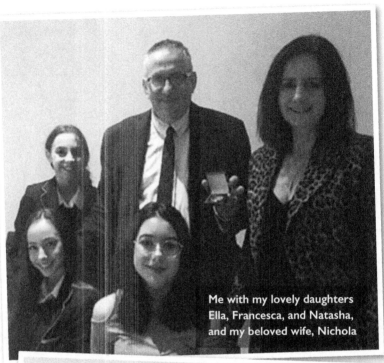

Me with my lovely daughters Ella, Francesca, and Natasha, and my beloved wife, Nichola

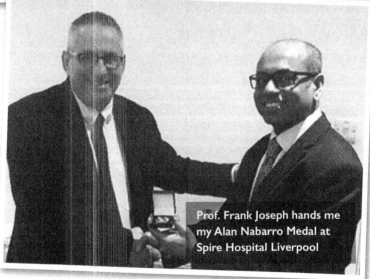

Prof. Frank Joseph hands me my Alan Nabarro Medal at Spire Hospital Liverpool

6
Life As A Legal Eagle

The life of a newly-qualified criminal solicitor isn't as glamorous as you might imagine, but I tried to do Michael proud. With the money grandpa Sidney had left me after his death, I bought my first sports car, a Triumph Spitfire. Yes, it was only second-hand, but it did the trick, apart from the day I went to Southport Magistrates' Court. When I arrived, I got out of the car, bent down to retrieve my briefcase, and heard a cartoonish RRRRRRIPPPPP! My trousers had split, all the way up the gusset, and were now flapping in the wind. I didn't have time to nip to Broadbents and Boothroyds for a pair of trousers, so I brazened it out. I went to court, and refused to take my coat off. The chairman of the bench said, "Mr Lee, are you all right?" And I said, "I'm sorry, Your Worship, I'm a bit shivery. Do you mind if I keep my coat on?"

I was just about to escape after proceedings, when a young lady lawyer of my acquaintance shouted, "Laurence! How lovely to see you. Do you fancy some lunch?" I didn't want to let her down, so I said, "OK, but I think I've got a cold coming on." And so I sat through lunch with this gorgeous young lawyer, who had no idea why I wouldn't take my coat off. I suspect she'd have run a mile if she'd seen what was beneath the coat. This sort of thing never happened to Michael...

I had to go to various magistrates' courts in those early days. Southport is now long gone, as is Crosby, which had a clerk called Mr Green, who was a very nervous man. If you gave him any kind

77

of problem, he'd go into a cold sweat and say, "I think we'll have to adjourn this. I can't deal with this this morning. Insufficient court time!"

But the main court was, and remains, Liverpool Magistrates' Court, though now it has moved from its old Dale Street premises to the Queen Elizabeth II building on Derby Square. When I first appeared at Dale Street in 1976, Rex Makin ruled the roost. But my favourite was Alan Berg, my legal hero, ever since I walked into No. 2 Court and I saw his unique style of advocacy. He would have done well on Radio 4's *Just A Minute*. There was no hesitation, no repetition, no deviation. His address to the court, his diction, was absolutely spot on. He reminded me of Patrick McGoohan from *The Prisoner*, who spoke in a similar way, with very clipped and precise language. I became very friendly with him. He was a very good joke teller, and I asked him if he would be my mentor. He agreed, and his advice came to be hugely important to me over the years.

Rex Makin was the lawyer I feared most, because Rex was daunting. He gave me no encouragement in court. One day I was in court, and Rex was behind me. I could hear his voice saying, "You shouldn't be appearing in this case." I ignored it at first, as he was clearly trying to put me off. But in the end I stopped, said, "Excuse me, Your Worships", turned around, and said to him, "Why shouldn't I be appearing?"

He said, "Because your boss's wife is on the bench."

"What are you talking about?!" I said. "It's three blokes!"

"No, your boss's wife is a magistrate, and so this bench is completely tainted."

While I was doing my articles, Rex was working in offices in neighbouring Hackins Hey, and I would often be given the job of taking post to Makin's. And when I went into his office, he had an old-fashioned window, and the window would open, like Arkwright's till in *Open All Hours*, and a hand would come out and grab the post. He wouldn't say thank you. He'd just growl.

We used to park in the same car park. And Rex knew my brother and his reputation. We actually got on well when we weren't in court, as I was no competition to him. I remember once walking along Exchange Street East, where Cyril's offices were, and Rex said to me, "How many paternity suits has your brother got out at the moment?"

I replied, "Come on, Rex, you're only jealous."

"Yes," he said, "I must admit I am." And in later years, he gave me an important piece of advice, which shaped my career.

When I started out, I looked around my colleagues and thought, "Who do I want to emulate?" Alan Berg was the obvious choice, but there was also Ian Levin, who was a former Lord Mayor. His command of the English language was second to none. I'd take a dictionary in with me, to check that he was using actual words. He would have done well on *Call My Bluff.* And, in fact, the standard of advocacy across the board in those days was excellent. Criminal law in Liverpool in those days was chock-full of characters. There was Malcolm Ross, or Mr Bojangles, the Ron Atkinson of the legal scene in Liverpool. There was Paul Rooney, who always had a pipe. On at least one occasion he put his pipe in his pocket and set fire to his suit. They were all characters.

At the same time, Robert Broudie, brother of The Lightning Seeds' Ian, and Julian Linskill were just starting out. There was a lot of competition. So it wasn't easy. Now, sadly, nearly every week I'm seeing colleagues dying or retiring, so the field is narrowing, and it's easier to get work. It's not so much because I'm good, which I must admit I am, but because there are few alternatives. "Oh, shit," clients say, "We'll have to instruct Laurence Lee now."

Julian Linskill had been a very good friend of my brother Michael. We all did our solicitors finals together. Prior to our final exam, Michael and I thought that we knew our conveyancing perfectly. Then Julian came round and said, "I say, chaps, can you quote Section 1 of the Law of Property Act?" Michael looked at me, I looked at Michael, and we said, "Piss off, Julian, will you?" Because he knew it and we didn't. And I think that for Julian, although he was to become a very well-known criminal lawyer, his best subject in his exams was conveyancing.

It was difficult for me as a young criminal solicitor starting out for another reason. I didn't exactly have a cushy life, having been a recently-diagnosed diabetic but I went to a private school and my dad was a GP. Quite frankly, I had a middle-class Liverpool background. The only time I ever really mixed with buckos - real Scousers - was at the match on a Saturday. I wasn't used to communicating with real Scousers, and it was a very rude awakening. In 1980, Liverpool celebrated its centenary of gaining city status. "Celebrated" is probably the wrong word. There was a Centenary of Liverpool festival at Camp Hill in Woolton - and it was a washout, mostly thanks to the weather. It was widely considered an absolute disaster. And the man who ended up carrying the can was Liverpool's director of education, Kenneth Antcliffe. He was pilloried, and was sacked by Sir Trevor Jones, the leader of the city council. But Cyril Carr, who worked with both men on the council, entrusted me with trying to get his job back. That's when I went on television for the first time ever, wearing a pair of glasses that were bigger than my face. Elton John would have been proud of them. And when I watched myself being interviewed on Granada Reports later that day, I cringed. I heard myself saying, *"Thar's only wun thing Mester Entcliffe wants, and thet's his job beck,"* as if I were delivering the Queen's Speech. And I thought to myself, "God, if I'm going to start doing criminal law, I'm going to have to change my ways a bit." And so I just got used to meeting so many run-of-the-mill, nice, down-to-earth people, that I changed my voice. I didn't exactly develop a Scouse accent, but I lost this very Received Pronunciation tone. And the glasses.

But I'd started going to the magistrates' court as a very raw 24-year-old, and at 24 it's very difficult to command the respect of criminals when you sound like Lord Snooty. So it wasn't easy to pick up good criminal work. But one day, I was standing around the magistrates' court and this bloke, who looked like a grizzly bear, a

Roy-Wood-of-Wizzard-type figure, came up to me and said, "Ey, are you a solicitor, mate?"

I squeaked, "Yes! That's me."

"Well, I've been watching you in court and I think you're f*****g brilliant, and I want you to be my lawyer."

That's an offer you can't refuse. So I represented him over the years for funny offences. For example, he was shoplifting in Chester one day, and, in order to escape, he took the drastic step of jumping into the River Dee, and swimming from one bank to the other. And when he got to the other side, the police were waiting for him with a blanket, because they liked and respected him. They took him to the police station, gave him a hot drink, and sent him on his way.

Unfortunately for him - and me - he told me one day, "I've got a case in Mold Crown Court tomorrow, and I don't want to go, so I think I'm going to pretend to have a bad back." So I said, "Well, I can't tell you what to do…" And then he was out in his car that night, crashed into a tree, broke his neck, and was killed. So that was the end of one of my best clients…

There are plenty of funny court stories from my early days. One of my favourites involved the guy who was arrested for not turning up at court. He was arrested the next day and the magistrates asked him, "Why didn't you come to court?"

He replied, "Well, I live at the top of a tower block in Everton, and I don't have a watch. I rely on the Liver Building's clock. And it was foggy, so what I thought was eight o'clock was actually twenty to twelve, so I was too late for court." The headline in the *Liverpool Echo* was "Misty Clock Proves Fred's Undoing".

Another chap did a similar thing, but when he was asked why, he said, "I'm schizophrenic." So I said to the court, "I think it must have escaped both of his minds." I'm not sure I'd get away with that these days.

I represented three generations of one family. The grandmother was an old-timer, a prostitute in Liverpool, the daughter was half-prostitute, half-thief, and the granddaughter stuck to thievery.

But the old dear was charged with biting a policeman's arm. She came to court and denied it. And when they asked her to give evidence, they said, "Did you bite this policeman's arm?"

And she opened her totally gummy mouth and said, "How can I bite without a tooth in me 'ead?" Case dismissed.

In the first big case I had, my client was a Chinese gentleman called David Lee, which was the same name as my father's. And he was up for counterfeiting currency. These were 50p coins, and they were so bad they wouldn't have fooled Stevie Wonder in a hurry. He was prosecuted and it went up to Crown Court, because it was a very serious matter, counterfeiting the Queen's currency. Prosecuting was a lovely chap called Michael Lee, which was the same name as my brother's. So we had a situation in which Mr Lee was prosecuting, Mr Lee was defending, and Mr Lee was in the dock. So when the magistrate said, "Stand up, Lee!" we all stood up, which caused hilarity in the court. Poor Mr Lee (the defendant) got a couple of years, because he produced a lot of these 50p pieces, even though they were shit. Why he picked 50p coins instead of £50 notes, I will never understand. You might as well be hung for a sheep, etc.

In 1981, my boss Cyril Carr, died after a heart attack. Cyril was on holiday in Rouen when he had the heart attack, but appeared to be doing well. He was flown back to Broadgreen Hospital in an air ambulance, but took a turn for the worse. He actually died next to Bill Shankly, his Liverpool FC hero. Cyril's death was announced in a newsflash on Radio City, because not only had he been a prominent member of the national Liberal Party, a former party chairman no less, but also he was, at the time, Lord Mayor of Liverpool. It was a tremendous shock to me, partly because he'd always been something of a hypochondriac.

When I heard the newsflash, I was with my ex-mother-in-law, Rosita Harris. She said, "It's terrible news." She waited a second, then said, "Congratulations. Buy that practice." My ex-wife, Lesley, whom I'd married in 1977, took a different view. When I went home to her, she was in tears. She said, "Cyril's died! You'll never get another job!" Lesley and her mother definitely had different outlooks.

Rosita - or Rose, as I always called her - really was my mentor in life. She would tell me exactly what to do, in business and otherwise. She had her own dress business and was breadwinner for the family. She was a fantastic woman and a terrific cook, especially for Jewish festivals and the Sabbath. But I had to seek advice as to whether I could handle all the pressures that this would entail. Had I not been a diabetic it would have been a definite yes. And, as I have always been determined that diabetes would never stop me doing anything, I made a decision: go for it. It was an example of my mantra: get busy living or get busy dying. Rose was right. I had to buy the practice.

It took about six months to get it sorted and deal with Cyril's mysterious representatives, who I never met. I was represented by his best friend, Gruffydd Evans, Lord Evans of Claughton, a lovely guy, and he looked after my interests, and we negotiated a deal. I also agreed to pay an annuity to Cyril's widow, Hilary, for 10 years.

At the time of Cyril's death, he was representing a Local Solicitor, who I won't name, in a Legal Aid fraud case. I took on the case after Cyril had died, but I had a £12,000 overdraft that was rattling up before I'd actually taken over the ownership of the firm and I desperately needed some funds. As you can imagine, £12,000 was considered quite a lot of money in 1981. But in 1981, although you had Legal Aid, you didn't put a Legal Aid bill in. The clerk of the court would weigh up your evidence and make the award of how much you were going to get. It was a system that was always likely to be corrupt. Luckily, members of the legal profession are upstanding examples of moral rectitude, and that sort of thing would never happen... So, at the end of this Legal Aid fraud case involving Mr Local Solicitor, I had all the files in some big whisky boxes, to pad the evidence out a bit. And I tootled down to the clerk, desperate for £12,000. The clerk said, "Ah, Mr Lee! You've got all the evidence there, have you? Yes, and a bit more, I suspect, as well."

"No, no, no!" I protested. "These are the case papers, sir."

His eyes narrowed and he said, "How much are you asking for?"

I gulped. "I think this is worth £15,000."

"Hmm," he said. "I'll give you £12,000 and not a penny more."

For the first and only time in my life, I was speechless, because I was so delighted and excited. And he said, "No! I know what you want to say. I know you want to argue and ask for more, but you're not getting a penny more."

What I actually wanted to say was, "I love you very much and I want to give you a kiss," but fortunately it never came out.

Cyril had three practices. When he died, there was Penny Lane, West Derby Road in Tuebrook, and Exchange Street East in the city centre. But immediately following Cyril's death the landlords wanted to treble the rent on Exchange Street East. After all, they no longer had a prominent city councillor and Lord Mayor there, and who was I? So I went to my legal mentor, Alan Berg, and he said, "What do you want town for? You don't need town. Go to Tuebrook and Penny Lane." And that is what I did.

The practice in Tuebrook was, before I arrived, a little backwater. We had one man there, who handled about four conveyances a week, and that was about it. But we had some real characters in the people I inherited from Cyril. These included a retired shipping director, Albert Lloyd, who was terribly posh and who became our messenger. Every Wednesday afternoon, he'd meet his old pals, one of whom was Billy Cook, who was Everton's full back in the 1933 Cup Final, which, incidentally, was the first FA Cup Final which had numbered players. Albert always wore a trilby, which he would doff and say, "Good morning, Laurenzio…" He always called me Laurenzio. And at Christmas luncheons, he'd always stand up and say, "I propose a toast to Laurenzio, the best articled clerk that Cyril Carr ever had!" What he didn't realise was that I was the only articled clerk that Cyril Carr had ever had.

We also had Colin Jones, who had been my immediate boss.

Cyril had had his first heart attack the month I joined, and Colin was the office manager. He was a very good conveyancer, but very much "of his time", which is the best way to describe somebody, shall we say, steeped in the mores of the 70s who indulged in antics that would be frowned upon today.

Six months after I joined Cyril's practice, I said to him, "Mr Jones, look, I've been on £10 a week since I joined. Is there any way you could have a word with Cyril and try to get me an increase?" And his reply was a sucking of teeth and an "I'll see what I can do." I never forgot it.

And then after Cyril died, I had become his boss. He came up to me and said, "I think it's about time I had a rise, Laurence. I haven't had a rise for a couple of years."

"Colin," I said, "I'll see what I can do…" Revenge really is sweet.

Colin was a very loyal servant and had been with the firm since the 50s. Unfortunately, he died in the late 80s after developing Parkinson's. He gave me good advice. For example, never accept first offers in accident claims. Or, if you get a letter that annoys you, never reply until you've calmed down. Just simple things, but these are lessons that you learn as a young lawyer, to just sit and reflect before you do anything. Never make decisions in haste.

Eventually, we also closed the Penny Lane branch. I had in mind the advice of Rex Makin. "Harrods," as he'd pointed out, "only has one branch." If it's good enough for Harrods, I thought, it's good enough for me…

Around the time of Cyril's death, when I was concentrating on criminal law, I said to my conveyancing partner, John Ablett, "Where are you going this afternoon?"

He said, "I'm going off to do a conveyancing completion at Gerald Strong's."

I said, "Are you?! Give me the papers. I'm going to do it."

So I went in there, to see Michael's old boss.

"What on earth are you doing here?!" said Gerald. "You don't know anything about conveyancing."

I said, "I know everything about conveyancing, Mr Strong." At best, I knew some conveyancing. He demanded a look at the paper.

He barked, "Do you realise this mortgage hasn't been discharged?"

I thought, "Oh, shit."

He said, "You'll have to draft a Discharge of Mortgage Form." So I agreed, and asked, "Can I have a cup of tea in the meantime."

Gerald, despite being Jewish, used to employ Arabic clerks, because he had so many Arabic clients, and was well regarded in the Muslim community. He had a young chap called Muflihi, whose family were respected and owned a shop in Toxteth. Gerald said, "Muflihi! Make Mr Lee a cup of tea. He's going to be here for some time."

So I drafted and sweated over this bloody document, regretting that I ever got involved. After about 20 minutes, I said, "Er, Mr Strong, where's my tea?"

And he said, "Muflihi?! Oh, the little sod's buggered off." He had as much control over his clerks as he did over my brother.

I never got my tea, but Gerald looked over the documents and said, "My God, it's right."

I'd drafted it correctly, and I thought, "Right, quit while you're ahead." And I never touched another conveyance after that.

That was one of the last times I saw Gerald. After Michael died, he was a broken man. He still carried on, but the last time I saw him he was in the Mercantile restaurant, where they did the most fantastic sausages, whatever they were made of, and he was sitting in a corner with two other men the same age as him, all probably late 70s/early 80s, planning to open up a new practice, like the Traveling Wilburys. They were starting a new practice the following Monday, called Elderly, Old & Ancient, I imagine.

Gerald died over the weekend before they were due to open.

The barristers I used were real characters. I think you have to be a little eccentric to be a good barrister. We've discussed Richard Isaacson before, and we will do so again. But one of my favourites was Michael Montgomery, who was a former BBC correspondent for Eastern Europe and who knew every Eastern European language. He was terribly "far back", in that BBC manner, and his humour was extremely dry. One of the funniest cases I ever had was with him.

It concerned an Egyptian sailor - let's call him Mr Hussein - who was accused of assaulting his step-child. He had a relationship with a lady of dubious repute in Belle Vale. And he was studying to become a merchant seaman. And the night before his exams, when he was studying in her flat, she went out on the town and made him look after her six-year-old son. But the child wouldn't shut up when Hussein was doing his studies.

And so, in accordance with his local culture, in order to shut him up, he held a heated knife towards the boy's face. I have to say I don't condone this practice, but I can see why you might be moved to it...

Unfortunately, and accidentally, the kid moved, there was a connection between the two, and he caused him a minor injury, for which he was accused of assault.

Michael Montgomery called him and me in for a conference. "Now, Mr Hussein, tell me about this woman," he said.

"Oh, Mr Montgomery," he replied. "Terrible woman. I was about to set sail from Grimsby after my merchant seaman exams. And the night before we set sail, she came on board and we made love. And three days later, the doctor, he diagnosed me with VD."

Montgomery, for whatever reason, said, "Excuse me, was that gonorrhoea or syphilis?" And Hussein said, "I don't know! He had grey hair and glasses!"

When I went into these conferences, because Montgomery's conferences were usually very dull, I always took my file, with an Echo folded up inside it so I could read the Everton story on the back page. Anyway, as soon as Hussain said, "...grey hair and glasses", my head disappeared into the file, and Montgomery's lip started twitching. And he said, "Th-thank you, Mr Hussein, and goodbye." And he kicked him out. He said, "Why on earth did I ask that question?" I don't know the answer to that, but I'm glad he did.

I have been involved in very few murder cases during my career. They sound exciting but they aren't. They're full of trauma, and on several occasions I've been threatened for representing defendants in murder cases. I'd rather have loads of drugs and fraud cases. It might be boring, but I like getting my teeth into a good fraud.

If I had a pound for every time somebody has asked me, "How can you defend somebody you know is guilty?" I could have retired 10 years ago to my yacht in the Bahamas. I always say this: the vast majority plead guilty, because if the evidence is overwhelming, I tell them so. I don't invent defences. And I tell them that if the evidence is strong and their defence is non-existent.

And, as a result of my advice, most will plead guilty. We have to advise them of the credit they'll get for an early guilty plea. If we don't we can get into ethical trouble. So we always advise about the merits of pleading guilty, and the vast majority do plead guilty. But on the occasion that people plead not guilty, even though we've tried our best to warn them that they've got no chance... be it on their own head. And I say to people, that in a democracy, everybody is entitled to a defence.

I love the camaraderie with my fellow lawyers and the judges. I think I've got humour, a pleasantness. Frequently, magistrates would say, "Ahhh, Mr Lee! Come and brighten up our morning!" And sometimes, as a bit of a joke, I'd stand in the back row, and say, "Just a moment, your Worships, I'm just going to go to the front row in case you can't hear me." I don't think I could ever be accused of being quiet, but I like to be pleasant, polite, humorous, and I'd like to think that I know my stuff... without being rude, that's the main thing.

But I also love the challenge of pitting my wits against judges, more so than magistrates, and prosecutors. I don't want to invent victory for a guilty client. But if they are innocent, I want to make sure that they're not convicted. And that's my challenge, to make sure that there's justice for the genuinely innocent. Some may say there aren't many of them, but there are.

I do all kinds of criminal cases, fraud cases mostly, all over the country, I do a lot of traffic cases - I specialise in helping people keep their licences when they get to 12 points. I've only lost one case ever. The important thing is that my clients are honest, and don't tell fibs.

I represented a lovely Indian doctor, who was a colleague of my dad's, and he kept speeding even though he was in his 70s, the Lewis Hamilton of the Liverpool streets. And he applied to keep his licence because he was one of those old-school doctors who did home visits, and his patients would suffer if he lost it. He told me that he would do eight or ten home visits every day.

He lost in the magistrates' court and appealed to the Crown Court. And I appeared before Judge David Aubrey, my old university classmate, and Judge Aubrey asked him how many home visits he did, and he said, "About two a month." He'd gone from eight a day to two a month. So if you're going to give evidence, give it consistently. If you chop and change, you're doomed. And he blamed me!

We also have a lot of historical sex cases ever since the Jimmy Savile scandal was brought to light. There are more and more prosecutions because, happily, victims are less scared coming forward. We have cases going back to the 60s. They're awful cases and upsetting, but again, somebody has to act for them. They're usually in denial, these defendants.

So I was slowly building the criminal law practice I'd inherited from Cyril Carr, despite my diabetes. But diabetes was always in the background, if I was lucky, and in the foreground if I was unlucky. From my first consultations with Dr Heinz Fuld, I had been warned about the consequences of eating too little, or over-exercising, or not eating within 15 minutes or so after taking my insulin. The symptoms of a hypoglycaemic episode vary from person to person and are difficult for a non-diabetic to appreciate. My symptoms were confusion, feeling hungry, and perspiring, and these symptoms still remain the same to this day. Thankfully, the warning signs last long enough for me to do something about it. To ignore these symptoms could be catastrophic, leading to fainting, and possibly could be life threatening. So I always carry a Crunchie bar or glucose tablets and after a few minutes I can literally feel my energy levels surging back to normal.

Only on one occasion have I bordered on losing consciousness. That was in the late 80s, when I delayed my lunchtime meal for what I thought would be a quick court case. Of course it took longer than expected and I began to feel dizzy and confused.

I came out of court in a daze though I still appreciated the need to get sugar into me as quickly as possible. However, instead of making me stop at the nearby kiosk for a Crunchie bar, my confused mind told me I needed a sausage roll for which I had to cross the very busy Dale Street. It's a miracle I didn't get run over.

The sausage roll didn't have the desired effect, so I ended up in casualty at the Royal Liverpool Hospital to get it sorted. I was due to fly to Austria the next day for a skiing trip. Although I was fit to travel, I felt the after effects of my hypo for days after, and my already pathetic levels of skiing sank to an even lower standard.

One of the most important years in my career was 1993. That year we represented some of the first people tried under the 1990 Computer Misuse Act. I represented a 22-year-old hacker whose handle was Gandalf. Along with his pal, known by the hacking community as Pad, my client had infiltrated machines running the UK stock exchange, the Ministry of Defence, NASA, and the Foreign Office. It was entirely baffling to me, but I had to go to interview with this young computer genius at Salford Police Station.

When I was at the station, it turned out that one of the servers he had hacked was that of the Joint Academic Network of universities, known as JANET. One of the questions at the interview was, "I put it to you that you have penetrated JANET." And I thought I was in the wrong room, for obvious reasons…

He was charged, and I said, "I suppose he'll be up at the local magistrates?" And they said, "No, he's in Bow Street." I thought, "Ooh, this is like Wembley for me." I'd never been to Bow Street, so I couldn't wait to get to Bow Street two days later. I went down there and was very disappointed at what a dingy and old-fashioned court it was. We were sitting in the corridor, and Gandalf said to me, "Have you seen Cleopatra?"

My interest was immediately piqued. I stared into the bustle of swots and brilliant boys sitting around at Bow Street. "Who's Cleopatra?"

He said, "Hang on, I think he's over there. Psst, Cleopatra!" And this spotty little Liverpool youth said, "Alright dere, Gandalf!" My God, Cleopatra? I was expecting Elizabeth Taylor.

Anyway, Gandalf eventually got six months in prison, but there were jobs lined up for him everywhere, because the universities wanted him to do work to safeguard their websites and computer systems. And the reason I got him in the first place was because his mum had once slipped on a grape in Tesco and we did the accident claim. Every little helps...

Also in 1993, we took part in the biggest drug importation case ever in Newcastle Crown Court, a case involving the notorious Curtis Warren. Our clients weren't involved with anything to do with importing. There were lead ingots in the back of a lorry and our client was allegedly in a car in front guiding it away from the main roads to take circuitous routes. As a result, we never got a mention for six weeks, which resulted in total boredom. And in the end the jury was so confused by who we were and if we were in it, it was a hung jury. Nobody had a clue. So they retried it later that year. But eventually we got him off.

Warren himself had a friendly bet with my barrister, Richard Isaacson, that he'd get off too. We bumped into him near WH Smith's on Allerton Road and he banged on the window of the car. "I'll bet you 50 quid, Rich, that I'll get off," he said. He did, too, that time, albeit on a technicality.

The case collapsed - and Warren supposedly burst back into

court to gloat to customs officers about his massive victory.

Sometimes, when cases are that complex, it's hard for juries to follow them. When we'd represented Mr Local Solicitor, who I shall continue not to name, for legal aid fraud, the barrister in that case was a lovely Lancastrian called Mick Maguire QC, a World War II veteran who was awarded the Military Cross. He always said to me, "In fraud cases you should always make the evidence as clear as mud to the jury." And he did. He completely bamboozled them. And in all the cases where we used him we won. The problem was that he used to confuse me as well.

But the most important case of 1993 - and the most important case with which I have ever been involved - changed the course of British history. It's the reason why I'm called upon to lecture young law students around the world, and probably the reason why you might have heard of me. And in the next chapter I'll explain exactly what happened when I was called upon to represent one of the two boys who killed James Bulger.

7
The Phone Call Of Fate

I was in the foyer of the magistrates' court on Dale Street when the call came. I had just been successful in a traffic case in one of the outer courts in Victoria Street, and it was too early to go back to the office. Besides, even though it was my firm, I was a terrible skiver in those days. So I decided to go back to the main court building, and have a cup of coffee with my pals in the solicitors' room.

I walked up the stairs to the main concourse, and it was packed full of restaurateurs and licensees. It was obviously licensing day and there were about 300 people in the foyer. You could barely move in the throng. At one point I turned around and went downstairs. Then I thought, "No, I'm not going back to the office. I'm going to battle through the crowds." Which I did. And I went into the corner of the foyer, where the solicitors' office was. There was a phone on the wall, and it was always ringing and nobody ever answered it. It was probably somebody phoning up to see if their lad had been up yet. But it certainly wasn't anything important…

Everybody on Merseyside who is old enough will remember vividly the news of the disappearance of James Bulger. James - never Jamie, despite what the national press might have called him at the time - was a two-year-old boy who had accompanied his mum, Denise, shopping at the Strand shopping centre in Bootle on Friday, February 12 1993. While she was in a butcher's shop, she had let go of his hand to pay for her shopping, then realised he had vanished, as little children often do.

There was a widespread search until his body was found by a

couple of schoolboys on a railway line near Anfield Cemetery, when the case became a murder inquiry.

Soon after the disappearance, police discovered CCTV of James being led off by the hand by two youths. The assumption was that the youths were young teenagers, and, in the following days, many of my colleagues had been called into police stations to look after boys who had been arrested. These had been playing truant on the day and were the original suspects. All of my pals had got such cases, and they were actually mocking me because I was the only one who hadn't. Frankly, I didn't really want to have one, because I'd promised my wife that I would never get involved. Of course, the reason I'd promised it was because it was a Bootle case and the chance of a Liverpool lawyer getting it was nil.

Anyway, for sport, God knows why, for the first time ever, I answered the ringing phone outside the solicitors' office in the foyer of the magistrates' court. The voice said, "You haven't seen Laurence Lee, have you?"

I explained that I had very recently seen Laurence Lee. Indeed it was I.

"Oh, that's a coincidence, aren't I lucky?" he said. It was Sergeant Bond at Lower Lane police station.

I said, "How can I help you?"

He said, "We've got a young lad in for the Bulger murder."

And I groaned, "Oh, no, not another truant?!"

He paused for a moment, then said, "I think it may be a bit more than that..." That was the understatement of the century. He continued, "Can you get down here as soon as you can? His mum's with him."

So down I went, to see what I can only describe as an angelic-looking boy. Jon Venables certainly did not look like the 10-year-old he was, he looked much more like an eight-year-old. I immediately thought, "He can't be involved in anything." The two police officers who were going to interview him, Detective Sergeant Mark Dale and Detective Constable George Scott, seemed very well trained in dealing with children. They had colouring books for him and as many bottles of Coca-Cola as he wanted and they made him feel at home.

It was an introductory interview at first. His co-accused, Robert Thompson, was being interviewed in Walton Lane police station, while we were in Lower Lane. And so young Jon gave his version of events. He explained that not only had he never been to the Strand, he had never even heard of it. Yes, he had been playing truant with Thompson, but they had been larking around in County Road, near Goodison Park, and that was it. And I thought, "I'm wasting public funds being here."

His mum, Sue Venables, was lovely, very polite and respectable. She told him, "I want you to tell the truth, please." And Jon said, "Mum, it is the truth. I've never been near the Strand. I was on County Road." As Brian Walsh QC later said, he was the most convincing little liar. He had me completely fooled.

After 40 minutes, we had a time out, and I was conscious that we should not have oppressive interviews, considering he was a child. After an hour, we reconvened, and I wanted this to be the last interview before the BBC's *Crimewatch* came on. That night, the programme was to show enhanced CCTV footage of the two youths leading James away to his death. DS Dale and DC Scott came back in and calmed Jon down with more colouring books and another can of Coke. And they said, "Right, we've been speaking to Robert. My colleagues have been interviewing Robert. And he says that you were in the Strand."

"No, we weren't!"

"Well, he says you were."

And then a silence and the moment I knew the walls were caving in. He said, "Well, we were in the Strand, mum, but we never grabbed a kid." He was wailing and hugging his mum, and even the officers. He hugged everybody except me.

And at that moment, I knew I was in for the long haul.

From that point he moved the goalposts from "We never grabbed a kid" to saying that they'd seen James, and then, yes, they'd walked him outside but they'd never done him any harm... and it progressed from there. I ordered the interview to stop at that point so we could watch *Crimewatch*. And the viewer could clearly see it was Thompson and Venables leading him out. And Jon was distinctive by his mustard-coloured anorak. I couldn't wait to get in the next morning. I burst in and said, "What colour is your anorak?" And he said, "Mustard." There was no doubt then.

That lunchtime, a Friday, I went back to my office to check that everything was all right. While I was there, Jon spoke to his mum, he called the police officers in, and he said, "I want to admit it. I did kill Jamie. Please tell his mum I'm sorry." I went back an hour later to be told this news and I had to endorse the custody record to the effect that this admission had been made in my absence and he had admitted killing, but not murdering.

Interviews after that became very torrid, and were about where they went and what they allegedly did. Sue, by now, had been replaced by her husband, Neil, a very nervous man. I told him that what was about to come out in interview would be awful, and he should just let it swim over his head. It was clear to me that Thompson and Venables had a hot potato, and when it got dark they didn't know what to do with him. Why they couldn't have let him go, and why the dozens of people who admitted seeing James with the boys on the two-and-a-half-mile walk from the Strand shopping centre to the railway line near Anfield Cemetery couldn't have intervened, we will never know. Finally, on the Saturday evening, Thompson and Venables were charged by Detective Inspector Albert Kirby, who was in charge of the case, and they were to appear at Bootle Juvenile Court on the Monday.

I was told I had to be there at 6am. So I got Angela Kauffman, my lovely and dependable secretary, to drive me there. Angela, who, sadly, is no longer with us, was like my mother hen and always kept me in check. She hated any kind of limelight and she said, "Make sure we're protected." So we drove up to the ramp under the court, having previously asked for it to be open. But it wasn't. So at six o' clock in the morning, we were waiting for this bloody ramp to open, and all the journalists who'd been getting an early pint at the Merton across the road were diving onto the bonnet, taking pictures. I loved it but poor Angela was mortified.

Eventually, we were allowed in and Angela disappeared. Jon arrived soon afterwards and we had our conference beforehand. And, when we were in court, he was remanded into the care of the local authority for a week. In those days, instead of just being sent up to the Crown Court, they had to have weekly remands. And, because I was going to go to court every week on it, a lot of my pals wanted to advocate on it. So I gave hearings to some of my dearest pals in the profession, all of whom were as experienced and competent as me. One was Paula Grogan, a friend of mine. She did one appearance for me. And various other people did a quick appearance, perhaps a five-minute appearance, not opposing the application, and adjourning for yet another week. I appreciate that this might sound callous or that we were treating a serious case like fun, but it's a part of the necessary distance that lawyers have to have from the content of proceedings in order to do our jobs properly, and to function from day to day. A big case is a big case, and lawyers naturally want to be involved, in the same way that a surgeon might want to be involved in a groundbreaking procedure.

And it is not as if the case did not affect me profoundly, even to this day. At the end of the first hearing, I had no way back to the office as Angela had left, and I looked out of the window, and I could see a baying mob. There were hundreds of people shouting "Let them go! Let them go!" like a football crowd. The police came up to me and they said, "Are you all right, Lol? You look a bit worried."

I said, "Can you blame me? Look at this mob!"

That's when they formed a scrum around me, and said, "You're a police officer, don't worry." So we went down the stairs, with me a hooker in this scrum, as it were. And they took me to Copy Lane police station, gave me a cup of coffee, and then they dropped me back at my office. The police were brilliant throughout, from the first moment of this case, utterly professional, but still with that combination of gallows humour and camaraderie that gets them through the day. I can't speak for the other lawyer in the case, who was representing Robert Thompson, but I had no relationship with him at all. Normally, in a case with co-defendants, you'd have some contact and cooperation. We didn't have any contact.

The baying mob did affect me, though, as did the fact that I was advised to check my car every day for bombs. It was stressful, especially after the arrest. I was extremely nervous and worried, and I remember feeling thirsty all the time, because the adrenalin really struck when he was being interviewed at the beginning of proceedings. And, of course, I wasn't sleeping well. My blood sugar was shooting up and it wasn't easy to get it down in those days. I couldn't just have a flexipen, as I would nowadays. I'd have to wait for the next injection and increase the dose. So I didn't feel great.

I needed help, so I phoned my mentor, Alan Berg. I said, "Alan, what am I going to do? I've had such a bad experience about the police station being cleared and the car being searched for bombs. I'm frightened of taking the case."

He said at once, "Don't be so bloody stupid. If you don't want it, I'll have it. Get in there." He was a really good motivator. And I was determined that nothing would stop me doing this case, least of all diabetes, as long as I kept an eye on my blood sugar. It just showed that nothing is impossible, despite diabetes. Nothing. And if anybody says to me, "Ugh, I'm not doing this. My diabetes is playing me up," they'll find I've got no sympathy for them whatsoever. Unless they're trying to get out of playing rugby at Liverpool College, of course…

I was still worried, because the public of Liverpool took it very badly. But one incident made me feel reassured. I was filling up my car with petrol on Queens Drive, and I was standing at the petrol pump. A big lorry suddenly appeared. And a trucker covered in grime and muck, who appeared about seven feet eight to me, clambered down from his cab. He said to me, "Ey, mate, aren't you that solicitor in the Bulger case?"

I squeaked, "Might be…"

He said, "I saw you on telly last night. I thought you were bloody brilliant. Keep your chin up." And that moment completely got rid of the worry and pressure. I got other messages of support, too. I wasn't one of those lawyers who proclaimed his innocence, or that it was a miscarriage of justice. I didn't blame the police or the public, I just got on with my job of representing Jon Venables. Every defendant is entitled to representation in a democratic society.

Eventually, Venables and Thompson were committed to the Crown Court, and the first appearance was in March at St George's Hall. At that point, I had to decide who would be our barristers. I had just finished the big drugs case involving Curtis Warren in Newcastle, and I would have wanted an unchanged team. But I was unsure about using Brian Walsh QC again. He had treated our 45-year-old alleged drug dealer, who was acquitted, very arrogantly. And I had no idea how he would be with Jon Venables, who was only 10.

Nevertheless, we had our first appearance in the Crown Court. Jon went downstairs to the cells and Brian was introduced to him for the first time. I was crossing my fingers that they'd get on. Brian said, "Hello, young man, nice to meet you."

Jon squeaked, "Hello, Mr Walsh."

Brian then took his wig off and put it on the radiator, and started trying to talk to Jon. But, instead of paying attention to Mr Walsh, Jon was paying more attention to the wig, and was staring at it intently. Eventually he said, "Mr Walsh, do you mind if I put your wig on?"

I thought, "Oh, my God, what's he going to say?" And he said, "Certainly, young man! Go for it!" And so there was a bizarre scene of Jon Venables, murderer of the century, wearing the QC's wig.

Jon was remanded to the care of the local authority for the duration right until the trial started, on November 1 1993, in Preston, and that's when we had to start taking proper instructions from him. But this was extremely difficult. After he had spoken at the police station, he clammed up. In those days, there were no psychologists or appropriate adults, and the hand of cards you were dealt was terrible. But we managed it in the end, thanks to my old friend Richard Isaacson. Brian Walsh was a stickler. He kept saying, "Oh, why can't you take instructions from this boy?" And I would say to him, "You've no idea how hard it is, because he's clammed up." Jon Venables always used to say to me, "You're not going to ask me any hard questions, are you?"

But Richard had a good idea. Both he and Jon had Nintendo Game Boys, and they both loved to play Tetris, the game in which you have to arrange falling blocks of different shapes into a wall. Jon, by now an 11-year-old boy, would have his Tetris, and Richard, a senior barrister, would have his own Tetris, and they would play with each other. Through this process, Richard would glean, like pulling teeth, little snippets of information. And I would sit in the corner with a notebook writing things down. It was terribly difficult to get instructions from him. But through that process he argued that Thompson was the guilty party. Thompson made him throw bricks at James, but he missed the toddler on purpose, and Thompson would say, "Are you blind, divvy?"

When they finally went to Preston, the Crown Court atmosphere was just unbelievable — so tense. Old men with cloth caps gawped at the sight of satellite dishes from the news broadcasters in the middle of Preston. It was alien, as if the spaceships had landed. There were 44 seats in the public gallery, and people would queue up from 5am to get a seat. And then, when Mr Justice Morland ordered the boys to be brought into court, I said to myself, "Savour this atmosphere for the rest of your life, because it'll never be repeated."

Managing stress throughout the trial was difficult. In those days, I had to have a jab in the morning before I set off. We stayed in a hotel in north Preston, in Garstang, and I used to have a normal hotel breakfast, and I was fine. I always had food with me. There was no blood-testing kit in those days. And I had to eat religiously every four hours. So I had to keep my eye on my diet, and the adrenalin from it meant I had to increase my dosage a little bit, because it was pushing my sugar up. I was running on adrenalin, so I wasn't getting ill, but I coped with it very well, considering I was diabetic. Of course, at that point I'd been diagnosed diabetic for 25 years, so I was a dab hand at it.

Jon's mother, Sue, was extremely stressed too, obviously, and I had to smuggle her out through the crowds to smoke outside. I was acting almost as a social worker as well as anything else. But in those days, I would be a very occasional social smoker, and pinch a fag, which was very naughty of me, being a diabetic. I must admit that I have, over the years, had the odd cigarette, particularly at Goodison. Mind you, watching Everton I've wished there was something stronger in there than tobacco. But when I used to go outside for a sly fag with Sue Venables, it calmed her down. And it calmed me down, because I needed it, because it was nerve-wracking. I would be too tired at the end of the day to go home, every day, though obviously I'd go home at weekends. But we'd go back to the hotel and chill out for a bit and have a nice afternoon tea to ease the stress.

Brian Walsh was exceptional in the trial, except for one thing: how he treated Richard Isaacson. Richard, God bless him, was determined to advocate in the Bulger trial. I'd advocated throughout the magistrates' court, so I'd had my fill. But Brian Walsh hogged everything. And even if it was just an application to the judge for half an hour remand, just to take further instructions, he'd do it. He wouldn't let Richard near. To add insult to injury, there was a court artist working for the media. You often see their pictures on the evening news, because it's illegal to make or take a picture of court proceedings. To get around this restriction, the court artist watches the scene, making notes, and then goes outside to draw from memory. This court artist drew this picture of Richard on his feet in front of the judge and it was pure fiction. He was furious about that, but also frustrated.

The trial ended on 24 November 1993, unexpectedly, at least to me. Venables and Thompson had also been charged with attempting to abduct another child at the Strand on the day of James' disappearance, and the foreman was asked to stand. "Have you reached a verdict on which you are all agreed?" he was asked.

"No," he replied firmly.

At that point I thought, "Oh, well, we'll be back on Monday morning."

But then, when he was asked if they'd reached a verdict on the main charges, he said, "Yes". I was stunned. The verdict was guilty. And Venables' mum wept discreetly. Thompson's, on the other hand, was furious. I won't repeat what she said.

Mr Justice Morland told Thompson and Venables that they had committed a crime of "unparalleled evil and barbarity... In my judgment, your conduct was both cunning and very wicked." And he detained them at Her Majesty's pleasure, later recommending a minimum term of eight years.

When the trial ended and I went back to my car, I got a call from a French radio reporter who worked for France Inter, Esther Leneman. She said, "What do you think about the verdict for Jon Venables?"

"Excuse me, Boy B, please," I said. During the trial, the boys, as minors, had been referred to as "Boy A" (Robert Thompson) and "Boy B" (Jon Venables).

"No," she replied, Jon Venables. The judge has just named them."

I could not believe it. I thought it was totally wrong and was very much against them being named. This was not so much out of loyalty to Jon Venables, but he had a young sister and brother, and parents, who were decent, respectable people. If he was named, they were named. So I said to a couple of reporters I was furious about the judge doing this, and thought nothing more about it.

A couple of days later, I was in London, and I was walking back towards Warren Street station, where I used to hang out, and I saw the billboard for the *Evening Standard:* Lawyer Slams Judge. I thought, "Who's been audacious enough to do that?" And I bought a paper.

Oh, shit, it was me! I hope he didn't find out, because I thought the world of Mr Justice Morland. He was a dignified, lovely judge, and very fair. And he was emotionally moved, as the jury was, by the content of the trial. I'm sure he had a tear in his eye at one point. And he had tried to keep the trial as child-friendly as possible, by the standards of the 90s.

A thunderclap like the Bulger trial, though, has echoes. Chiefly of course, there are echoes for Denise Fergus and Ralph Bulger, James' parents, who have behaved with such dignity after their unimaginable loss. Denise, particularly, has done so much good in the name of James in the years following his death.

There were echoes for politics. Tony Blair, who was Shadow Home Secretary at the time of the trial, gave a speech in which he said, "We hear of crimes so horrific they provoke anger and disbelief in equal proportions... These are the ugly manifestations of a society that is becoming unworthy of that name." This became part of his rewriting of Labour's position on law and order, and became part of his platform when he replaced the late John Smith as leader of the party and, eventually, as Prime Minister.

There were echoes for the law. Lord Chief Justice Taylor raised the minimum sentence to 10 years. And the Conservative Home Secretary, Michael Howard, in a naked bid for electoral popularity increased the tariff to 15 years. The increased minimum term was overturned by the House of Lords in 1997, which ruled it unlawful for the Home Secretary to decide on minimum sentences for young offenders.

Richard Isaacson had said, with great foresight, "In years to come they will call this trial unfair." And in 1999, the European Court of Human Rights held that it was an unfair trial. Not unlawful, but unfair. So proceedings for juveniles in the Crown Court are now less formal. For instance, if the Bulger trial were happening today, the judges wouldn't wear wigs. And they certainly wouldn't have a trial in Court No. 1 at Preston, which was a horrendous court. I went back there in 2020 for the first time and I saw Court 1 and I almost burst into tears, it was so emotional. It brought it all back. Because there were echoes for me too.

At one point I did start to feel the strain and I needed a few days away from the pressures that I was in danger of buckling under. Before 1993 I had rarely been on television or radio, but now my comments were in demand all over the world, especially after the trial had concluded.

I must pay tribute to my dear friends Noel and David Glover, who have a cottage up in the Welsh hills, far from the madding crowd. They'd seen me on television and feared I wasn't looking well and they offered me the chance to get away from it all for a vital respite break.

Although I'm a townie, it was amazing to spend time where mobile phones hardly work and the only views are rolling hills and farmland. Noel and David offered me sanctuary and I will be eternally grateful to them - they are my adopted brother and sister.

And I had nightmares after the trial. I was so mentally strung-up by it, I kept having the same recurring nightmare about being run over by a ghost train, which I suspect was connected to the train which ran over James' broken body. And I didn't get rid of that dream until I went skiing with Richard Isaacson the following February. I think the Alpine air got rid of it. Or perhaps the fear of breaking every bone in my body in a skiing accident.

I've always been more protective of my own girls than maybe I would have been, had I not been so closely involved with the Bulger trial. I remember, even before I had children, after the case had finished, I went with my friend and his son to see Everton somewhere in the Midlands. We stopped at a service station, and my pal said to his son, "Go and get some sweets from the sweetshop, will you?" And I screamed, "No!" And went with him, because I was so scared that he could be kidnapped. I became neurotic.

My relationship with Jon Venables, however, is most certainly over. We kept in touch with him for about six months, because he and Thompson started appealing against the Lord Chief Justice and Michael Howard's increase of the tariff. But when there was a suggestion that it was about to go to the European Court, Brian Walsh said to him - and we all agreed - "Every time you speak to us, you're looking backwards. You've got to look forward now, and, therefore, you really need new lawyers." And that was the end. In 1994 we said goodbye, and I've never laid eyes on him since.

I'll never understand why he did what he did. Albert Kirby, the police officer in charge of the case, and some of the other officers think he and Thompson were born evil. I don't believe that. I think they were born into difficult backgrounds, which is not sufficient reason, and opportunity knocked and they carried out evil deeds. I don't think they were inherently evil. I always say that if these boys had been born in the South of France, or somewhere more middle class, it wouldn't have happened. You had to have all the ingredients to be in place at the same time. It was a toxic brew of circumstances and opportunity.

But this case never dies. There are always anniversaries, and people come back to talk to me. It's always coming back for Denise, poor James' mum. And it lives with me, never diminishing. I was recently at the Old Bailey, and even the QC said to me, "When we next meet, I have to speak to you about the Bulger case."

Even so, I do welcome the opportunity to talk about the case. I've always loved press coverage, although I had a rude awakening, as far as that was concerned, because of the very first time I did a radio interview on the subject. I was downstairs in the office, and Angela, my secretary, said, "There's a radio station wanting to speak to you. They're on now and want to do a live broadcast." So I rushed up three flights. And I gasped, "Hello!" I was so out of breath. And so I did a live interview that sounded more like an advert for Ventolin inhalers. So I knew that I either had to lose weight or get fitter before I did any further interviews. Or do them on the ground floor.

In 2000, the BBC asked me to go to Norway to interview the mother of Silje Redergård for the *Correspondent* programme, which was presented by Edward Stourton. Silje was a four-year-old girl who was killed by two boys aged five and six in Rosten, near Trondheim. This programme was to contrast the approach to serious juvenile crime in the UK and Norway. The Norwegians treat children who have committed crimes very differently. There is much more of an emphasis on rehabilitation and almost none on retribution, because children under 15 cannot be prosecuted.

I flew to Oslo Airport from Manchester, hours late, after the thickest fog I had ever seen had cleared. I felt as if I were in a spy novel - *Tinker Tailor Soldier Solicitor*, perhaps. I was excited and had my insulin with me, but the delay made me worry about what food would be available. I always had an emergency pack with me - biscuits, a banana, and, in those pre-9/11 days, a bottle of Lucozade. We got into Oslo Airport at about 9pm, and the building was shut. I had no idea how I'd get to Trondheim that night, but I found one little office at the far end of the airport that was still open.

They sent me on a bus to a hotel nearby with a view to catching an early morning flight to Trondheim the next day. After I had arrived at the hotel and dumped my bag in my room, I went back down to reception.

"I've never been to Oslo before," I said. "Can you get me a taxi for Oslo, please?"

"Sir," the receptionist said, "this is Oslo Airport."

"Yeah, but it can't be far…"

"It's 80 miles from here," he said. I can see where easyJet and Ryanair got their ideas from.

The nearest town was 30 miles away, so I went back to my room and, as there was no food on offer, I raided my emergency package. It was a good job I brought it.

The next morning, I flew into Trondheim to meet the producer, Guy Smith, who went on to become a BBC Home Affairs correspondent. Guy told me filming would start at 11am at Trondheim railway station, where I would walk from the train as if I'd arrived by train. He was an absolute stickler. I had to coincide my script with the opening and closing of the automatic doors. I got trapped twice. It was about Take 17 when I finally got it right.

Eventually I spoke to Beathe, little Silje's mother. She was not angry with the two boys who killed her daughter. She said, "They were nice little boys. They used to sit on my knee." I couldn't believe her attitude. I felt like saying, "Get a life, woman. This is crazy. Why weren't they locked up?"

But I spoke to the chief of police, a Spurs fan called Terje Lund. He said, "You can't incarcerate kids. It's unheard of in Norway." And everybody I spoke to thought we were inhumane in England, with an age of responsibility of 10. It was such a different society. If I opened a law practice in Norway expecting to represent criminal juveniles, I'd have been bankrupt in a week.

I always wanted to go back to interview Silje and see if she had changed her mind, but never did. However, *The Guardian* spoke to her a few years ago, and now at last she has feelings of anger.

I've spoken to people around the world about the James Bulger case, aided by the fact that I speak French and German, although my interviews were often so bad they had subtitles in that language, which is a bit embarrassing. Once I was having lunch in the car, eating a sandwich, when the phone went and it was Abbe Smith, who was a law lecturer at Harvard. She said she'd heard about the case, and asked if I would be prepared to come over and give a talk to the students. It took me a microsecond to agree at some stage to come and do it. Subsequently, she moved from Harvard to the American University in Washington. So I had a lovely week in Washington at cherry blossom time, and it was just beautiful.

I had one friend in Kathmandu and he saw me on telly there. I went to my favourite hotel in Zermatt and the receptionist said, "Oh, Laurence! You've been on Swiss TV every night this week." It's been a great buzz, but the novelty wears off.

And once I had a case in France, a Scouser who was arrested on an international warrant in northern France, and, because I spoke French, he abandoned his normal lawyer for me to represent him in France. So I instructed Jean Boully, the father of a friend in France. Professeur Boully was the equivalent of Rex Makin, only more pleasant, if you can imagine such a thing. He was a really great guy and also lectured bar students. He said to me one day, "Come and meet my students tomorrow at 9am." So I went in and saw these students, and greeted them in my rusty French. And he said, "Maître Lee was involved in the Bulger case and he will now talk to you for 20 minutes about the Bulger case *en français.*" The swine! So I asked the students, "Do you speak English?" I received not a word in reply. Nobody claimed to speak any English whatsoever. And so I began addressing them in broken French, and there was a word I needed. I couldn't remember the French for "case", which is fairly important when it comes to talking about the law. I said, "What's the French for 'case'?" And this guy said, "I think the word you're looking for is *procès*." Perfect bloody English! So they made me go through the rigmarole of going through a lecture in pidgin French. I reminded myself of the English policeman in *'Allo 'Allo*, "Good moaning, I was pissing your ship."

But what it's taught me primarily is that diabetes couldn't stop me from handling the most serious murder of the century. A lot of people might have thought, "Hmm, I'm going to embark on something stressful here. I don't think I'm quite up to it." And a lot of diabetics might have felt that way, especially newer diabetics, who haven't got the confidence that I've managed to accrue in 50 years.

But what I say to them is "If I can do it, you can do it. There's nothing brilliant about Laurence Lee, apart from a few letters after his name, but there's no reason why, and I know it sounds corny, you can't embark on any aim that you have in life." I climbed the legalistic version of Mount Everest, I played at legal Wembley, and it made me very very proud of myself. And a quarter of a century later I'm still here.

8
My Blue Heaven

On Tuesday, 17 April 1973, Everton were due to face Chelsea at Goodison in the league. Normally, that would have been a cause for celebration for me and my dear dad, David. But we were Jewish and that was something of a sticking point.

You see, in 1973, Passover began on Tuesday, 17 April. It was the tradition that we would have two dinners on the first and second nights of Passover, called Seder. We would have boiled eggs with salt water and matza as part of a tasty, slap-up meal. It was a night full of old rituals.

So my dad and I were perturbed to notice, about a month before the game, that it would take place slap bang on the first Seder night. I said to my dad, "Look, much as I love the Jewish religion, I'm not missing the Chelsea match." And it wasn't even as if we were any good in those days.

But what were we going to tell grandma Edith and grandpa Sidney?

We tried writing to Everton to see if we could get the date changed, but there was fat chance of that. But my dad had a lot of connections within the club through his job. He was doctor to various people at Everton. And, probably as a mark of respect to him, they invited me and my dad in to meet the club secretary, Chris Hassell.

Chris said, "Look, we're very supportive of the Jewish community, obviously." Of course, back then, Liverpool's Jewish community was much bigger then than it is now. He went on, "If you give us the list for next season of all the Jewish festivals, we'll try and make sure that no match takes place that day." Of course it was nonsense, but it was nice of them to indulge us.

So we had done our best, but the match was to go ahead with Everton and Chelsea on the Seder night, and I told my grandmother, who'd prepared her usual fantastic dinner, that, unfortunately, I had to revise for an exam the next morning and I wanted my dad to test me on the exam.

And so, off we went to Goodison. We left the match a few minutes early - out of guilt, mostly - and we knocked on Edith and Sidney's door, when they were just about to serve dinner. My grandmother was serving the food, and she said in her broken accent, "End how vas the studying?"

"Oh, very good, thanks, Grandma." She waited a moment, then struck the killing blow. *"End who scored the vinning goal?"*

My cover was blown, and it was frosty for a few weeks afterwards, but I put Everton first and I don't regret it.

And who did score the "vinning goal"? It was Howard Kendall. If you had told me then that I would end up drinking in a Formby pub with Howard some 30 years later and helping to organise his testimonial, I'd have had you sectioned...

Sidney died later that year and Edith died in 1980. My mum died in 2010, and my dad died the week before the FA Cup Final in 1995. And he'd have been at the match too.

He wasn't born an Evertonian, but he became one, and he was almost as fanatical as me. He died on the 50th anniversary of VE Day, with his medals next to his bed. On the night of the shiva prayers following his death, Everton were still fighting relegation, just before the Cup Final, and they were playing Ipswich away. The rabbi was leading the prayers when Everton scored. And suddenly there was a shout, "One-nil!"

Everybody said, "Shh!"

The rabbi said, "Quiet...!" Then he said, "Who scored?" It was

Paul Rideout, for the record, and that was the night they became safe. Thanks, Dad.

Ever since that first match in 1965, when my dad was given tickets out of the blue by a patient, one of the biggest things that's kept me going in life is Everton Football Club. Everton has been my pressure release valve. It was my aim to go to my first match after becoming diabetic, that fifth-round FA Cup match against Tranmere. And my aim then became to go to Wembley later that year for the West Bromwich Albion final. I still can't forgive Jeff Astle for his thunderbolt, God rest his soul. So Everton have lived with me and I've lived with Everton ever since. All my holidays, even my first honeymoon, revolved around when Everton were playing and where they were. I've had a season ticket since 1970, and I had missed fewer than a dozen games before the Covid-19 pandemic. During that pandemic, I missed more home games than I had in my whole life up to that point. I had been there for every league match, every FA Cup tie, every European night, every disappointing League Cup tie, every possible conceivable match, even those which made me wish I were elsewhere in freezing temperatures... I'd like to think they have helped me control my diabetes by releasing stress and I do feel better for it. They've always been my lifeline, even though they've given me a lot of heartache over the years.

Because it was love at first sight with Everton. I remember smelling the tobacco in the air as my dad and I walked towards the ground, because back in those days, people smoked pipes, besides cigarettes. There was this intoxicating aroma as we approached the ground and one could see the floodlights getting nearer and nearer. For a kid of 11, it was magical. These days, the smell of the tobacco going towards Goodison has gone, replaced by the whiff of sausage rolls and onions on burgers, which has its own appeal for somebody at my age and with my waistline.

My official connection with Everton started in the early 80s, with my work with the Everton Shareholders' Association. I enjoyed working on that committee very much, and was there for many years. In 1984, as a result, I was invited to the FA Cup Final banquet at the Lancaster Hotel. I took my parents with me. I suppose it was a way of paying back my dad for introducing me to one of the great loves of my life… and my mum for indulging us both.

Shareholders' Association meetings were always interesting. I was deputy chair for a while. And I was there in 1995, following our FA Cup Final victory over Manchester United. I sat through one meeting with the FA Cup right next to me. I couldn't keep my hands off it. It was incredible, and I'm just sorry my dad didn't get to see it. The Shareholders' Association was a very old gentlemen's committee. It was taken over in a coup in 2003, and I didn't want anything to do with that. I stormed out, as the Liverpool Echo put it at the time, along with Professor Tom Cannon. It was a real military coup. A load of new shareholders, who had never been to the annual meeting before, just swarmed in and voted out the chairman and his deputy.

I suppose a lot of people thought we were just taking advantage. For example, we would be in a ballot to be in the directors' box. But I always hated being in the directors' box. I'd much rather be in my own seat. And they thought we were too cosy with the board. But that was the point. We reasoned that we needed to be close to the board, because the more cooperation we had with them, the more we'd get out of them. As they say, you catch more flies with honey than with vinegar. I'm glad to say, though, that to this day, the small shareholders have managed to stay independent and not be taken over by club owners. It's important that supporters retain a voice, as our friends across Stanley Park are beginning to appreciate…

At school, I was in the same class as Glyn Jones, the son of Sir Trevor Jones, the Liberal councillor and occasional rival of my future boss, Cyril Carr. Glyn was an Evertonian - and I used to say to him, "Do you think we'll ever meet Brian Labone?", because his dad knew Brian Labone. And he said, "No, chance." Back then, I was praying to meet Joe Royle and Alan Ball and the rest of the team. They were like gods to me, golden and immortal. Of course, I never did. But that began to change when I went to the Hawthorns to watch Everton playing West Brom in the Third Round FA Cup tie in 1989. It was the first time the two teams had met in the cup since the 1968 final, and, before the match, they wheeled out the surviving members of the 1968 cup winning team. I looked at them and I was shocked. A few of them were using sticks. One of them was in a wheelchair. It was obvious that their career had taken a heavy toll on them. I thought, "If they're like that, I wonder if the Everton players are the same."

It preyed on my mind, and some time later I received a phone call from David France, the chairman of the Everton Former Players' Foundation. If there were a Premier League of football fans, David would be top every season. David instituted the Gwladys Street Hall of Fame, collected a staggering amount of Everton memorabilia, and had created Blueblood, which became the Everton Former Players' Foundation. I knew him through my work with the Everton Shareholders' Association, and he asked me if I'd be interested in joining the foundation. I said I'd be delighted to, but I insisted on bringing with me my dear friend Richard Lewis, who had served with me on the Shareholders' Association. He is also the greatest dentist on earth.

It was a great organisation. The foundation was self-sufficient, and we had it in our articles of association that any player who had played one senior match since the war was entitled to help. So we started out helping out for orthopaedic needs. We paid for wheelchairs, we'd pay for hospital care, if it wasn't NHS. We'd always pay for operations especially for new knees and new hips, because when they were playing, keyhole cartilage operations did not exist. They used to use cortisone injections, and the effects were terrible for the players. And then, in later times, if a player died, we'd pay for the funeral. Even after that, we would look after the widows. Pat Labone, our administrator - and widow of the great Brian - puts on monthly lunches for the Everton widows, or the Toffee Ladies, as we call them.

We would have our meetings at the Adelphi Hotel, in the grand surroundings of the boardroom there, before we had them at Goodison. But David became ill some years later and he asked me to succeed him as chairman. He said, "I'm not retiring unless you take over." So I had to. And I did it for 12 wonderful years.

And why wouldn't I? I mean, why wouldn't I enjoy going to a meeting at Goodison Park? I have the same thrill going on a Thursday night at 6pm for a meeting as I do going to the match. Even more so if it were during the Mike Walker era...

The club has always suggested that they take us over, but we've always insisted on our independence. Of course we're very great supporters of Everton In The Community, but I don't want us to become part of them, even though they're magnificent. But the Former Players' Foundation has to retain its independence to keep its focus on the former players.

Our main fundraising events have been dinners. We used to have dinners at the St George's Hotel and we've had them at Goodison as well. We always have a Christmas lunch for the Former Players' Foundation, and we get around 70 former players. I always invite my dear friend John Keith, the broadcaster best known for his work at BBC Radio Merseyside and Liverpool's City Talk. He's a surprisingly good impersonator of people. Harold Wilson, Ted Heath, Bill Shankly, Bob Paisley. And he knows all the former players, Fred Pickering in particular. I'd always thought John was a Red, but he's actually a big Wolves fan. But he followed Liverpool through Europe in the 60s, and has great stories about Shanks and Paisley, but this book is not the place for stories about the Reds. It would be sacrilege.

At the end of every season, the club allows us to use the pitch, so we have an annual Play On The Pitch Day, and that raises so much money, because people are desperate to play on the pitch. They come out to *Z-Cars* and they have Everton kits and we get the likes of Graeme Sharp and Graham Stuart to be manager. We even get proper referees in and have awards in the 300 Club.

I'm glad to have been able to give something back to my idols, in their time of need. But I'd be lying if I didn't say that I've loved the opportunity to get to know these heroes of mine. Even though I deal with judges and high-ranking members of the legal community, I have less fear standing up in front of them than I do in meetings with former players.

One of the treats we've given former players is taking them to the pantomime at the Theatre Royal in St Helens every year. And so I have a fond memory of walking down Corporation Street in St Helens, where the theatre is, sharing a bag of chips with Brian Labone. Harry Catterick called him "the last of the Corinthians". He'd won the league twice, and the FA Cup, and only missed out on playing in the 1966 World Cup because he was marrying Pat. And now he was eating chips in St Helens with me. Take that, Glyn Jones! By then, Brian had become Type 2 Diabetic. And he said, "Make sure, Lol, we don't tell our specialists we're having this bag of chips." He was a lovely guy. He used to say one Evertonian was worth 20 Kopites.

I also got to know Gordon West, Everton's legendary goalie of the 60s and 70s. I'm not a great autograph hunter, but I've got six autographs by Gordon West. Every time I used to see Gordon, he'd say, "Do you want another autograph?" So I just collect autographs by Gordon West. Gordon used to moan to me about modern players' wages, and I can't blame him. Of course, when he was playing, when I was a kid, players were paid fairly well, but they were still very much in the community. They might have owned the nicest house in your street, but they still lived in your street. Things are very different now. Gordon would say to me, "£100,000 a week? If I were playing now, I'd play for a month and pack in." Brian Labone told me once about how they were paid in the 60s. For every 1,000 attendance over 30,000, they'd receive an extra pound. When Brian and Gordon came out onto the pitch, Gordon would say, "Hey, look, Brian, there must be 55,000 out there. That's an extra 25 quid!"

Gordon died in 2012, and at his funeral at Liverpool Cathedral, I was invited to recite Psalm 23 from the pulpit, which was the greatest honour.

Gordon would agree that the namby-pamby players of today are a totally different breed. I had a cartilage operation and soon after Bill Kenwright had put on a production at the Empire. My darling wife, Nichola, and I went to one of the performances, and afterwards we were in the lounge and I came down the stairs on crutches. And Jimmy Harris, who played for us in the 50s and 60s, said, "Hey, mate, what's the matter with you?!"

I said, "Well, I had a cartilage operation last week."

He said, "In our day, you'd be out for the season if you had a cartilage. It's bloody keyhole now, isn't it?"

"Er, yes, it is."

He said, "Throw your bloody crutches away and come with me to the bar."

And out of sheer embarrassment I said to Nichola, "Just hold these for me, will you?" And suddenly I could walk. A miracle! Jimmy took the Mickey out of me, and was saying to the other players, "Hey, he had a cartilage operation the other week and he pretends he can't walk!" How embarrassing!

I was very friendly with Dave Hickson, the only man to play for Everton, Liverpool, and Tranmere Rovers, though Everton was his true love. He used to say, "I'd break every bone in my body for every club I played for, but I'd die for Everton." He had a heart attack, years before he actually died, on the day we beat Southampton 7-1. And when he woke up a few hours later, the first thing he said was, "What was the final score?!"

One of the great things about Dave was his answering machine. It said, "Sorry I can't take your call. I'm just rearranging my quiff."

I also met Alex Young, the Golden Vision. He was a lovely guy too. I met him in Goodison Road in the main office, near the lifts. We entered the lift together, and I said, "Which floor would you like?" And he said, "Would you believe the Alex Young Lounge?"

Where else would he be going? I felt such an idiot.

I've got to know Gordon Lee, our manager in the late 70s and early 80s, through the foundation. He comes to the Former Players' Christmas meal most years. He has a very dry sense of humour, but is a good man. I had met him years earlier, when he was manager at the Feyenoord match. To get into the changing rooms at the ground there was a ramp that used to go up, and Gordon was a bit late and banged his head on it as it came down, so that he sported a black eye at the airport. Bob Latchford hadn't played in that game because he was on strike. And I said to Gordon, "What's the problem with Latchford?"

He said, "The problem with Bob Latchford is he wants to live in Southport and play for Barcelona."

I helped to arrange the testimonial of Gordon Lee's successor, Everton's most successful manager and one of my boyhood heroes, Howard Kendall. I used to meet him in his pub in Formby. I have no idea how I ever got out alive. While we were arranging his testimonial, I went out to see him and I parked my car for five minutes. And he was having a little drink. I joined him and, inevitably, I was with him for an hour and a half and I got a ticket. But it was worth it. He was so entertaining, but he was never drunk. I used to see him every Christmas at Ken Dodd's lunch for the Good Turn Society. And, during every lunch, all his empty white wine bottles were turned upside down in the ice bucket. We used to call them his Dead Soldiers.

My favourite memory of Howard is after Everton won the FA Cup in 1984 and were in the European Cup Winners' Cup. The first round was against University College Dublin, and I went with the team to the away leg. It was moved from their ground to a bigger ground, which was still only about the size of the old South Liverpool ground in Garston, and the tickets were like wedding invitations. One of my friends and neighbours was Howard's dentist, Clive Layton. And, at the beginning of the second half, Howard said to Clive, "Can you just look at this filling?"

And so there was this bizarre picture of Clive, looking into Howard's mouth as the second half was about to start, and him turning round and saying to me, "I can declare that Howard is dentally fit." And then we carried on with the match. We were lucky to get through that dour 0-0 draw away. Luckily, the great Graeme Sharp scored in a 1-0 win at home, and Bayern Munich and Rapid Vienna awaited.

So I've met many of my heroes, but Joe Royle is my No.1. Or, I should say, my No.9.

I'd met him before, when he was manager, but I hadn't got close to him. But we became instantly mates when we were on the committee. I always call him No. 9, and he'd still be on the first team if I had my way, even if he has got dodgy knees. He's a legend. That word is overused, but it's exactly what he is. Joe's got such good connections with the PFA that they make a big contribution to whatever medical costs we have. And Joe's in constant touch with them and was very supportive when I was chairman. And at the end of each meeting we'd have such fun telling stories about former players.

I was chairman for a long time. I felt like Robert Mugabe. I was re-elected by a show of hands in 2015. But by 2017, it was becoming less of an old boys' club. People had joined and they were more hands-on with sick players. And, of course, I was in court every day. I couldn't give it the dedication I should have done. So I was voted out by half a vote - an abstention - and, really, looking back, I should have been delighted.

I'm still a trustee, ex-chairman, and am very supportive of the current chairman, Henry Mooney. We've got a fabulous committee, and my biggest allies are Joe Royle and Pat Labone. At first I think people thought there'd be sour grapes and I'd throw my dummy out of the pram, but I said, "No, I will never leave you, even though I've been voted off. Unless you tell me to go." And Henry is very respectful of me and my experience. So, I've got no jealousy. I'd served my time and dedicated 12 years to being the chairman, and loved every minute of it.

Besides, it was through being chairman of Everton Former Players' Foundation that I embarked on one of the most rewarding, if surreal, periods of my life. I'd been chairman for a while, and then, in 2005, I received an email, which I assumed was a wind-up from one of my play-acting friends, purporting to be from Barcelona Football Club, asking me if I'd be interesting in helping them form a European Former Players' Association.

When I eventually phoned the signatory to this email, it turned out if was no joke. It was from Ramon Alfonseda, who was a sort of utility striker for Barcelona. He was like Mick Bates of Leeds, or Alf Arrowsmith of Liverpool, the best reserve going. Bill Shankly had told George Scott, "You're the 12th best player in the world." So Ramon Alfonseda was probably the 12th best player at Barcelona. And he was the chairman of their former players. He invited me over to their initial meeting, their initial congress, of EFPA, which was to take place in Sitges, the Jewel of the Mediterranean. And we were treated like royalty. There were representatives from former players' clubs from all over Europe. There were two little old men from Bruges, there was a chap from Bayer Leverkusen, another from Real Madrid. Funniest of the lot was the representative from the Russian Federation, who couldn't speak any English, except for "Let's cha-cha!" He just wanted to go out on the town, as if he'd just climbed over the Berlin Wall. He contributed nothing. The meeting was going to be Sunday morning, and he never turned up, presumably because he was pissed. But we were taken on guided tours of Barcelona, with police outriders in front of our coach, and plied with the most fabulous food. And I felt as if I were acting under false pretences getting there.

Eventually we had our first meeting on the Sunday morning, and they said, "How are we going to create a European Former Players' Association?"

I said, "Well, can I just speak from what we do at Everton?" Because we were unique and played a big part in the meeting. I said,

"We have a database of about 1,000 former players - if that. Can you imagine the size of the database for Europe? It must be hundreds of thousands. There's no way you'd be able to fundraise to make money for them. Therefore, the best way to do it would be to seek the help of UEFA."

Now I knew this would never work, and it was pure bull, but I said, "Why not ask UEFA if they would donate a euro cent from every Europa League - or UEFA Cup as it was then - ticket, Champions League ticket, international matches? And if we got that euro cent, that would make a lot of money." They thought it was a very good idea, so they formed — and I was embarrassed — a subcommittee of Everton, Barcelona, Real Madrid, and Bayer Leverkusen. And I thought, "God, please one day let that be the semi-final line-up for the Champions League." It hasn't happened yet, but it might. I went home thinking, "What a bluff merchant."

But a few weeks later I had a call from Ramon saying, "Can you come to Geneva next week?"

I said, "What for?"

He said, "We've got a meeting booked with UEFA."

Shit! I said, "Yes, of course I will."

So I got tickets to Geneva on easyJet, and we stayed in a grand hotel. The next morning, a big black limousine came, with UEFA flags fluttering off the bonnet, and we were taken to Nyon, and my feelings never subsided. I think they call it imposter syndrome. We arrived at the glittering UEFA building in Nyon, and it was all made of pinewood and glass and marble and overlooking Lake Geneva. We went in, and I was hoping to meet Lennart Johansson, the UEFA President. But we met Lars-Christer Olsson, who was the number two. And we went in there. He said, "Very good of you to come, gentlemen. But Laurence, I owe you an apology."

I said, "Why?!"

He replied, "I am afraid the view of Mont Blanc is shrouded in mist today."

I said, "Mr Olsson, can I tell you? I work in a place called Tuebrook. We pray for fog."

He laughed and said, "Help yourself to souvenirs." I've still got the UEFA pen. And they even invited me — because it was the year Everton got into the qualifying round of the Champions League — to the draw. I didn't go. I think I'd have probably smashed the place up when I found out we were playing Villarreal. It still rankles! Barcelona invited me as a guest to the away leg, which was really lovely. "Go to the box office and there'll be tickets waiting for you."

So we walked into the meeting at UEFA headquarters, and Ramon was the spokesman. I was just sitting there with my mouth open listening to all of it and just enjoying the atmosphere of it. He set out all the aims of the Former Players' Association. And he mentioned that we were going to have games in aid of homelessness, Kick Out Racism, and the usual causes. But he said we wanted primarily to look after former players and do what we could for them.

And Olsson looked at us through his steel-rimmed glasses. He said, "Gentlemen, you remind me of a hunter that goes out into the forest in the middle of the night with his rifle and he takes 20 random shots, and he goes back the next morning to see if he managed to hit a bear." He told us, basically, that our plans were slapdash, but it was a good idea, and they gave us a really big financial donation.

He said the idea about tickets was basically old hat, if they'd had a euro cent for every time somebody had suggested it they'd be millionaires. It was bullshit on my part, but it was a good start. And it resulted in enough money to act as a Zip firelighter for the organisation. It paid for congress and we had a lot of people going to the first annual congress.

The following year, they wanted me to speak about what we do at Everton. And there were translators there. There were hundreds of people in the audience. The next guy who was going to speak for Barcelona Former Players was a chap I'd never heard of before, but I got chatting to him and he seemed lovely. His name was Pep Guardiola. No idea whatever happened to him…

There was a little man sitting at the front of the congress, and I was telling them what we do for our old boys, about all the funerals and the healthcare. This chap stood up and said, "I want to congratulate you for everything you do for Everton former players." And I realised he was Alfredo Di Stéfano, the Real Madrid legend. I couldn't believe it. I nearly cried.

And I met so many big names. We put on a charity match for tsunami relief at the Nou Camp between a Shevchenko XI and a Ronaldinho XI. When I went for meetings at the Nou Camp, every three months, I'd just sit in the stand at the stadium and look at it, reading that motto "Mas que un club," over and over.

Before the tsunami match, we had a meeting and there was a knock on the door, like Skinner and Baddiel used to have on *Fantasy Football League,* and in walked Sepp Blatter and Lennart Johanssen. Blatter totally ignored me, but Johanssen said to me, "I'm so grateful to you for coming all the way from Everton." It was classy of him.

Now, on the way there, at the airport in Manchester, I was wearing my Barcelona badge. The tsunami relief game was a very well-publicised match, and there were quite a few people going to the game. A chap came up to me and said, "Are you going to the match tonight?" He was too, but not in the directors' box. I nodded.

He said, "Do you think Johan Cruyff will be there?"

"Oh!" I said, "I've never given it a moment's thought. I suppose he might be…"

He said, "Well, if he is, can you get his autograph for my son Jack? He's only 11, and he loves him." His son Jack had never heard of him. It was for him.

It was the coldest match I'd ever been to, including at Goodison. And we were in the directors' box, and I couldn't wait to get in at half time for a hot drink. When we got to the door to the directors' lounge, on this marble floor, there were waiters dressed in black suits and bow ties, serving up malt whisky in a lovely goblet… just like Goodison, really. With pie and chips. So I said, "Have you got anything hot?" And they gave me a bowl of chicken soup.

So, as I'm thawing out with my malt whisky and my chicken soup, guess who's next to me? Now as I said, apart from Gordon West, I'm not an autograph hunter. So I said to Johan Cruyff, "Look, this is very embarrassing, but…" — and I felt like a weirdo because I said, "I'm very friendly with this little boy…" — "would you mind finding a piece of paper and a pen and putting your name on it?" And he wrote him a little letter. He said, "It would be my pleasure." And he wrote, "Dear Jack, I wish you well…" and went on.

When I got back to Manchester, there was the dad. He said, "Did you manage to get the autograph?" I said, "Yes, I did, actually."

"Oh, Jack will be delighted!" he said. And he took it off me and shoved it straight into his top pocket.

But one of the best times I had was in 2006. The night before the Europa League final, wherever it was, the plan was that we would arrange a veterans' match of players from Europe against a team from the host country. So the final that year was in Eindhoven. Middlesbrough were playing against Seville, and so they wanted to arrange a match of a Euro XI against a Dutch XI of former players. My job was to find a coach for the Euro XI.

One of my best friends, Jonny Dexter, the Liverpool optician better known as Jonny Goggles, was very friendly with Sir Bobby Robson. Sir Bobby had sat on his glasses at Anfield at midday and broken them, and Jonny had a new pair for him by 1pm. That's how Jonny Dexter is. He said, "Why don't you try Bobby?"

So I got his number and Sir Bobby messed around. First he was Yes, then No, a bit like when he was once about to become Everton manager. He dithered. My wife Nichola, even though she didn't like football, used to call him The Ditherer.

Then I remembered that one of my friends in London was very friendly with a chap called Dave Butler. Dave was the physio for England, and a very close friend of Terry Venables. Wherever Terry went, Dave went. The cogs turned in my brain. So I asked Dave Butler, and I mentioned it to Ramon, and I got in touch with Terry, and he said he'd think about it. Then Ramon phoned him and, as I was driving back to the airport from Barcelona, Ramon phoned me, very excited. He said, "I speak to Terry. He agrees to do it."

So Terry became our coach, and it was such fun having meetings with him. I met him a couple of times in Barcelona, and, of course, having been manager there, he knew all the restaurants. As a surprise, we got Steve Archibald to come with us. Steve was his big mate and favourite player at Spurs. Everybody loved Terry. So I said I wanted Dave Watson to come from Everton. I insisted on having an Everton player... If I was there, if I had anything to do with it, he had to have an Everton player. And I was very friendly with Dave Watson in those days.

So Terry agreed. And then he said, "I didn't know you meant him! I thought you meant the long-haired bloke from Sunderland!" We got Ally McCoist to play. We had some great players, Thomas Ravelli in goal and Gheorghe Popescu. And the Dutch team had the Van Der Kerkhof twins, who owned a restaurant in Eindhoven. We ate at their restaurant after the game, and Terry saw these guys, who were a bit chubby, and he said, "These two look like a pair of librarians."

Anyway, we beat the Dutch XI 3-0, and I was allowed to sit on the bench at the Eindhoven training ground. And I wanted to sit with Dave Watson and Ally McCoist at the meal, but I had to sit with the committee on the grown-ups' table, which was a shame.

It was a great night, but it never happened again because the whole thing went bust. We had all these congresses, and then gradually they wanted to expand more and more and they became too big. And I kept warning them they were expanding too much. It was like we were trying to take over the world. Unfortunately funding ceased, and that was it. And I was really annoyed because it could have been a good thing. While it was small, it was viable. And it had UEFA support, but I think they thought we'd grown too big for our boots. There was nothing fraudulent about it, but I think the problem was they were building up publicity to such an extent that the publicity used the funds that should have gone to help the former players. But they did create a lovely former players' lounge at Barcelona, and I'd go in there and see the old boys playing chess. One day they said to me, "If you come tomorrow morning, all the old boys will be having a practice kick around." And I went to this complex where there were about six synthetic pitches, and they said to me, "On this pitch, they are over-40s. On the next pitch, they're over-50s." And I saw these guys over 50 just standing behind these little goals, and one of the guys said to me, "There are six European champions playing here." In spite of their age, their skill was just fabulous.

Then we went to the little restaurant where the footballers and training kids go. They have a school there for the kids, and all the kids were having lunch, and we were taken into an ante-room. The chef came out with his black-and-white chequered apron and said, "What would you like?"

I said, "I'd love a steak." And they made me the best steak I've ever tasted. I don't think Scouse pie was on the menu…

I was invited to another lunch at Barcelona. They were going to play Real Madrid the following Saturday, and I was sitting with the directors of Barcelona and the representative from Real Madrid was at the other end of the table and they hated each other. The history is frightening. And they were chatting away, and the guy from Barcelona whispered in my ear, "I hate these f***** bastards."

I became friendly with the representative from Bayer Leverkus-en, Michael Kentsche, who used to play for their reserves. In fact, I was the only representative there who wasn't a former player. Just purely a fan. Michael was obsessed with cricket, even though he'd never seen it played. And when we were at the airport, he said to me, "Laurence, we have two hours, teach me the rules of cricket." Two hours?! You need two weeks… I was just about to embark on the LBW rule, when he looked at me and said, "Shit! My plane leaves in five minutes. I must go!" So he never did find out.

Other teams in the UK have tried to set up associations similar to Everton Former Players' Foundation, but they rarely work. Liverpool's former players' association is lacking. I used to speak to Ian Callaghan and David Fairclough and people to try to get together and have a joint meeting. But it never materialised. But it's frustrating, because every club must have supporters who can afford to assist. I was in contact with a solicitor who was a Man United fan and was keen to start a former players' organisation, but it's all organised by players. We're the only ones who are run purely by supporters.

I do believe that it says something important about Everton, that it's the fans who run the Former Players' Foundation. David Moyes got it right when he called it The People's Club. It's important because we can look from the outside at what the needs of the players are. I think players may not look at it from the same viewpoint. Again, in Europe, we were the only club made up of supporters. It was great seeing former players from other clubs, but it wasn't the same.

The only club that was anywhere near us was Glasgow Rangers. They had a fantastic guy called Colin Jackson, who died recently. He was part of the team that won the UEFA Cup in the 70s. His testimonial was against Everton. But sadly, everywhere in Europe, West Brom, Everton, they're human and they're mortal. And day by day, I feel sympathy when I see the likes of Ian St John and Tommy Smith die. And all the players of Leeds — my second club — who've died recently. And every week we see somebody who's passed on, Nobby Stiles and so many of the 1966 England team. Thank God Joe Royle is only young at 72. We've got to keep them in cotton wool!

I have been fortunate through my involvement with the Shareholders and the Former Players, but I've always been wary of exploiting my involvement with the club. I hate encroaching, because even though I was deputy chair of the Shareholders' Association, and then chairman of the Former Players' Foundation, I never wanted to take advantage of anything I could get. Because I could get whatever ticket I wanted, because one of my dad's patients was the lady in charge of the box office, so we would always get good tickets for Everton, and by 1985, we were on the front row of the Main Stand, where I still am today. We used to sit next to Derek Hatton. I used to get on well with him and he's a mad Evertonian. I remember we scored against Liverpool in the derby and he lifted me up - because he was a fireman, of course - and he said, "Ahhh, this is better than sex!" I think it was a reference to Everton scoring. I hope so, anyway.

But I think part of the reason I like sitting in the crowd, rather than up in the directors' box, is because it means I'm the same as everybody else. And that's been the aspiration of my life, to show that having diabetes doesn't single me out as special. If I manage it properly, I can do the same as anybody else.

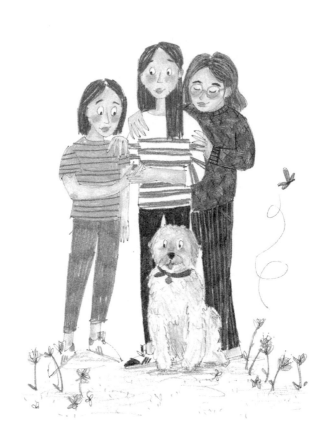

9
Get Busy Living

In 1994, not long after I ended my involvement with Jon Venables and the Bulger trial, my father, David, was heading towards the end of his life. We actually shared a consultant at that time. My hero, Dr Heinz Fuld, had long since retired, and both my father and I were under the care of Brian Walker. Dad had heart problems and had developed Type 2 diabetes in later life, which meant he too needed the services of an endocrinologist.

He was in Lourdes Hospital, on Greenbank Road, close to the synagogue we used to visit, and I visited him every evening after work. On one particular day, I was later than usual, due to an over-running court case, and I dashed into the hospital to get to my dad before he had his supper.

As I entered the hospital, I passed a huddled-up old man, who was being helped along by a younger woman. I stopped a few moments later. There was something about this old man that I couldn't place, so I turned back to see who he was.

It was my hero Heinz Fuld, along with his wife, Pat.

I went up close to him and said, "Is that you, Dr Fuld?" I could tell that his eyesight was failing.

He replied, "Is that you, Laurence?"

"Yes," I said. I could feel my eyes prickling.

He said, "I saw you on television, Laurence. I was so proud of you."

I burst into tears and hugged him.

That was the last time I ever saw my life-saver and eternal hero, but I did receive a letter from him in which he said that, at 98 years of age, he could only walk 50 metres and needed a magnifying glass to read.

He died in January 2008, 40 years to the day after he diagnosed my diabetes.

Brian Walker was a lovely man, but he wasn't strict enough with me. I could go years without having a specialist appointment, and so my blood sugar wasn't properly monitored. I'm convinced that I'm lucky I have good genes. An average diabetic, if he hasn't had his blood tested for years, will have all kinds of complications over the years, and I haven't. My mum, Hazel, was a poorly controlled diabetic, and she managed to avoid complications, as did my grandad, Sidney, and I think they've passed that down to me. Of course, I was able to test my own blood, but it wasn't as easy in those days as it is now. I would have to go down to the hospital to have my normal blood tests and then find out how disastrous they'd been.

I started with Brian Walker in the late 70s, but I drifted. He was a fabulous and kind man, and he was looking after my dad till he died in 1995. So he'd come to the house, or I'd see him walking in the park when I had my cocker spaniel, Oliver, but he'd never ask me about myself. What he lacked in the scientific side of things, though, he made up for with his bedside manner. When my dad was very ill he'd come in and say, "Hello, David! Oh, I love these paintings." My dad was mad about his oil paintings. There were so many of them, we had to store half of them in the loft, and it drove my mum to distraction. He had a patient who was an Irish art dealer. My late brother had very little faith in this man. We had a balcony in Casa Blanca, my parents' house, and one day Michael was standing there, looking out at the world, and he said, "Oh, God, that bloody art dealer crook's arrived!" loud enough for that bloody art dealer crook to hear. He couldn't care less.

My wife's best friend, Debbie Jones, was a pharmacist married to a heart specialist called Mike. And he asked me, "What is your

HbA1c?" HbA1c — or Haemoglobin A1c —measures how well controlled your blood sugar has been over a three-month period. I felt very uncomfortable being quizzed about my condition, knowing full well it was probably bad, but Mike sent me to Whiston Hospital to see one of his friends for a blood test. And, of course, when the results came back, they were, to say the least, not good. And that's when my wife, Nichola, said, "You've got to go and see somebody who's going to give you a kick up the arse like you deserve."

That's when Dr Jiten Vora came in. He was the opposite of Brian Walker. He was all stick and no carrot, and that's exactly what I needed at that time. He'd test my HbA1c, and in those days my score should have been five. And once he said to me, "Six is shit. Eight, that you're on, is DEATH."

I said, "Well, when do you want to book the funeral?"

He said, "You've gotta get it down."

He'd test my blood pressure when I went to see him. He'd say, "Your blood pressure's too high."

I'd say, "How can you tell?"

So he'd use a blood pressure monitor — PUMP, PUMP, PUMP — and then he'd show me.

"Oh, it's too high?" I'd say, "You know white coat syndrome? You give me that. Every time I come in here, I shit myself."

He told me, in the most forceful of terms, that I had to change from animal to human insulin. He would say, "This insulin you're on is shit. Why don't you change?"

I said, "I will change, I will change…"

He said, "There's always some excuse. It's either Everton, or you've got a case in London. I bet you you will want to change."

But I didn't want to change over at first, because I hated change. As Howard Kendall would tell you, you don't change a winning team. It got to a stage at which I spoke to one of my dad's best friends, Murray Kirwan, who was the police surgeon and a very well-known figure in Liverpool at the time. I told him I was desperate to carry on with the animal insulin. And Murray went round all the police stations in Liverpool, into the fridges, and got me the final stock of animal insulin, and I carried on with that for as long as I could.

But then I was feeling pretty rotten, and I realised I had to bite the bullet. So I phoned Vora, and said, "Look, you've won your bet. I want you to book me into Lourdes Hospital, just for the night, and I'll tell you when I'm going to do it. Everton are playing Portsmouth a week on Tuesday. I'm going to go to the game, then I'll come straight to Lourdes. You can change me over, and see how we go."

So I popped in after Everton had played Portsmouth, and went to bed with a nighttime jab of Humulin, the artificial human insulin. I woke up next morning and had my breakfast and said, "Ooh, I feel OK, actually. I think I'll just stay here for the day."

"You must be joking," he said. "You're out. Have your breakfast and bugger off."

He was right, of course. I was fine. I was better than fine, actually. I hadn't felt that good since I was a kid. I'd been running at third gear at best, and now I was comfortably on fourth gear, even overdrive, where I've largely remained. That's thanks to Dr Vora, who was a taskmaster at least as tough as Heinz Fuld. He used to batter me during our sessions, and then, five minutes later, he'd be asking me if I could pass him any cases so he could make some money out of medical reports. He was tough, but he was a good guy and he meant well. Mind you, I was pleased when he retired.

Following that, I settled on my current specialist, Professor Frank Joseph, and he is absolutely magnificent. He's easy going, but firm at the same time. He keeps me happy, because he's so upbeat and positive. He says he's proud to have me as a patient, and he is so supportive. And out of all the specialists I've had, I think he's right up there alongside Heinz Fuld. Blood sugar testing took three days in the time of Dr Fuld. Then I went onto the blood pricking test about 10 years ago, which took about half a minute. Now Prof.

Joseph has attached a sensor disc, about the size of a two-pound coin, to my arm. I wave it in front of my phone, and I can receive a whole graph showing me where my blood sugar is in a micro-second. What a huge difference! Diabetes when I was a teenager and diabetes today are totally different. Insulin is so much better, and monitoring my condition is so much easier. There are times now, especially when my blood sugar's good, that I feel I could sprint. And there are times in the park, when I'm with the dog and the girls, that I have sprinting races with the girls at the age of 68, because I feel so good. I used to need to be motivated by hard taskmasters like Dr Vora and Dr Fuld, but they've trained me in such a way that Frank Joseph doesn't need to treat me like that. He's happy with my progress. He just says to me, "Let me see your phone." The only problem is that I have to change my sensor every two weeks, and it's like pulling an Elastoplast off my hairy leg, which isn't great fun.

Really, the advances in modern science, along with things like Everton, and satisfaction with my job in spite of stresses, have kept me well. But it's also been the support of friends and family, particularly Nichola, who used to bully me about it, "Go and get your HbA1c tested, for God's sake! Get your prostate checked!" She was absolutely fabulous, and that's something I'll miss.

Because I lost the love of my life in December 2020, after a long battle with her own illness. I met Nichola Evans through my connection with Paul Feather, the hotel chain owner. When my brother Michael died, Paul became my client and she became his PA. We got together a few years after my divorce from Lesley in the early 90s. I'd often see Nichola and she'd be in my office every day. But she never had any interest in me whatsoever. I'd ask her out for coffee, but she'd be far too busy. In the end I clearly wore her down. She told me later the reason she didn't want to go out with me was because my shoulders were too narrow.

But we became soulmates, and after a couple of years it was clear we were going to be married. So I decided to take her to a country pub. And while she was getting ready to go — she always took a long time to get ready — I wrote a poem for her in order to propose…

> The smell of cow shit in the air
> Makes me dream more than I dare
> Of life with you and total glee
> For Pete's sake *[her father's name was Pete]*,
>   will you marry me?

I inherited poetry writing, if you could call this poetry, from my mother, Hazel.

Nichola made me get down on one knee in a puddle in the Alvanley Arms in Cheshire. It was worth it. We married on 1 September 1999 at Coombe Abbey, a hotel Nichola had found. It was a reformed monastery from the 13th century, and all the staff were dressed as monks and friars. The theme of the wedding was "Merriment Aplenty", and it really was. And in the following years, we had three daughters, first Ella, in 2001, and then the twins, Francesca and Natasha, in 2006.

After she left Paul Feather's firm, Nichola worked for the council, in charge of inward investment. She was responsible for getting Coutts Bank into Liverpool, among other big companies. And it was only when she went on maternity leave with the twins that they shafted her. So she took redundancy and she was at the school playground when she and her future partner, Andrea Edwards, who had worked at McDonald's as a manager hatched a plan to go into catering. And so they opened up the Interesting Eating Company on Allerton Road. They never looked back. Nichola and Andrea opened up restaurants all over the country with JD Sports, who wanted eateries inside their shops. They were going to go for one of the big names. But Nichola went to see them and said, "Why don't you try us, because you'll love our food?" So they went to the Interesting Eating Company, sampled the food, loved it, and in no time they were opening up 10 food shops specialising in pancakes in places like Nottingham, Preston, Kingston upon Thames, and Rotherham.

She wasn't always that good at sales, mind you. I was dating Nichola when my father died, and my mum said, "Look, we've got to clear out some of your dad's paintings. I'll tell you what we're going to do. There's an art auction down in Eastbourne. Sotheby's. I want you and Nichola to go down to Eastbourne for the weekend and get rid of some of these bloody paintings."

So Nichola and I had a lovely weekend at the Grand Hotel in Eastbourne. And on the Monday morning off we went to the auction. It was a novelty. I'd never been to one before. We were given a paddle, watched the other people holding up the paddles, all the bidding… It was great fun.

Anyway, when we came back to Liverpool, my mum said, "Right, you had six paintings to sell. How many have you got left?"

Nichola proudly announced, "Seven!" She'd seen a picture she adored, of a lovely sleepy Arab village, and none of our paintings went at all. They didn't even reach the reserve price. But she had to bid 200 quid for another bloody oil painting. Mum went mad.

Nichola was just my rock, and very supportive in business. If anything, she was too intrusive into my business. I used to say, "Look, you've got pancakes to sell. Sod off and let me defend criminals." Uli, my German friend who had always encouraged me to reach for the heights, and Nichola got on like a house on fire. He just loved her. And since her death, so many people have told me how much they adored and respected Nichola.

But sometimes people say to me, when they hear I've lost Nichola, "I know how you feel." The fact is they don't know how I feel. I'd lost my brother and I'd lost my parents, and those losses were tragic and very upsetting, especially my brother. But I never thought losing somebody could be like this. Even though Nichola was ill for many years, it still feels like being hit by a train. She was a few years younger than me and had only just turned 60 when she died.

She was diagnosed about three years before her death with Parkinson's Disease. And, for a year, you'd never have known anything was wrong. We went to Disney World and walked miles. It was only when we went to Spain for half-term that I noticed in the airport that she was shuffling and didn't look right, and it went downhill from there. Her mobility went. My poor wife spent months in different hospitals. And in the end, it turned out that she didn't have Parkinson's at all. It was more like a motor neurone disease. And it debilitated her completely.

Poor Nichola. Her illness was like the sea coming in on the beach. The water kept lapping up, so she would go backward to keep away from the waves. But it was relentless, and in the end her back was against the sea wall. This book is dedicated to her. I'd been planning to write it for ages, and she would say to me, "How are you getting on with this bloody book? Get on with it! Just go in the other room and write the damn thing, instead of watching stupid Everton!"

Oh, yes, she hated football, with a passion. I don't know what she did to deserve being married to a fan like me. She used to find out the result before I got home to see what mood I'd be in and prepare for it. And she was even less keen on dogs than football, but that was a battle she managed to win until near the end. We got Alfie while Nichola was ill. She always said, "I'm allergic to dogs." Was she hell?! When she was very ill we found out she wasn't allergic to dogs at all. She was allergic to horses, just like my brother Michael.

So we decided during the Covid-19 lockdown to try to find a cockapoo. Alfie's a bit bigger than a cockapoo, but she finally relented as long as we got a dog that didn't moult. So we went down to Nottingham to pick him up. Nichola was extremely poorly in bed all day long, being looked after by her carers. The girls and I brought this pup upstairs and said, "There's your little friend, Alfie." What were her words?

"Take him away! He stinks!"

Anyway, she did get closer to him, and he used to lie on her bed. I think he was a comfort and companion in her last days. And, since her death, little Alfie has plugged a massive gap, especially for the kids. They adore him.

Nichola's death was a tragedy, and the sort of devastating event that could easily have screwed up my diabetes. But, as the district nurse said, "Look, the last thing you want is to get ill with young children." And Nichola would have gone mad with me if I'd allowed it to affect my health. So life had to go on, and we had the most fantastic carers that came in during the day before things got really bad. They got her dressed in the morning and to bed at night. One in particular, Harley Morrison, only 25, became the best of friends with Nichola and the plan was she would become Nichola's PA. She would take over insurance on the car, take her shopping, take her to the hairdressers... I'm sure Nichola would be delighted that our multi-talented Harley ended up illustrating this book and is still a close family friend.

Harley was devastated when she died. In fact, she was with her when the dreaded moment arrived. I missed out by five minutes because of bloody Everton. I'd spoken to Nichola that morning and I said, "Look, I'll come over straight after the Burnley/Everton game." And it finished at 2pm. I set off straightaway, and she'd died just about then. The timing was unexpected, if not the death itself. One love of my life kept me from the other in the end, I suppose, but if anybody would have understood, it would have been Nichola.

The funeral was tinged with some humour, though, because the rabbi who taught me my bar mitzvah, Norman Zalud, who's now 84, conducted the service. I wanted him to do it, so I wrote him his speech, and paid him a fortune, and he kept calling Nichola "Monica". And at the end of the service he said, "Rest in peace, Ella." Ella's my daughter's name. And Ella shouted, "I'm only 19, for God's sake." The place was in uproar. Nichola would have loved it. She'd have said, "Soft sod." He phoned me the next day and asked if there was anything else he could do. "God," I thought, "You've done enough damage already." The girls converted to Reform Judaism, and he taught them Hebrew and Jewish history. Nichola herself wasn't Jewish, she was Anglican. But Nichola became a Friend of the Synagogue — though she didn't convert — and so she's buried in the Reform Jewish cemetery, close to our home.

But, in spite of all this, I had to carry on. I don't mean I had go to work straightaway, but I had to make sure I wasn't ill. I'd seen it coming — she'd been ill for so long, her death was no shock. And yet it was the finality of it all. But I made sure I ate. Jane Johnson, our housekeeper, has been a fantastic support. She has kept the girls together and has been like a second mum. She insists that I eat well and don't let it get me down, because I'm now the girls' rock. Nothing is going to stop me being well, certainly through diabetes.

I've always made sure that I've stayed on the straight and narrow, without being a boring sod like grandpa Sidney. I've never been a clubber, but I've minimised excesses. A little bit of what you fancy does you good, as they say, but I've never taken drugs, apart from two spliffs in university. I used to have the occasional cigarette when I watched Everton, but I've cut that avenue of pleasure off as well, to Nichola's delight. I'm not a big drinker. I like a glass of red wine. When you're diabetic, you should have everything in moderation. It sounds a bit dull, but I'm determined to live as long as possible, subject to being knocked down by a bus. But, for the sake of the kids, I've got to keep myself in cotton wool. But if you do that too much, you stifle. You suffocate.

And so, outside of work I have turned my hand, admittedly to a pathetically low standard, to football, skiing, tennis, and golf. It therefore came as a delightful shock when I was honoured in 2009 to be elected captain of my beloved Childwall Golf Club.

I have to say that it wasn't my golf skills that persuaded the powers-that-be to appoint me, but that I could always spin a jolly good yarn. This meant the members of Childwall could laugh at my stories as well as my golf. Golf captaincy involved playing matches on a far more frequent basis than I'd ever been used to and I had to adjust my diabetic regime. Eighteen holes of golf without a buggy involves a several-mile walk, even if you hit the ball straight. Yours truly, of course, would hit the ball in all directions, resulting in a vast increase in the distances I had to cover. I had to decrease my insulin intake and arm myself with loads of sugary goodies such as Lucozade and Mars bars to fend off the threat of hypos. I also took with me my trusty blood-testing kit to make sure I was on the straight and narrow with regard to blood sugar.

Over the whole year I managed my diabetes very well, because I brimmed with self-confidence. I could easily have shied away from taking on golf club captaincy, but, again, it was a question of getting busy living or get busy dying.

Diabetes was never going to stop me from achieving any of my dreams - it never has and it never will. The downside was the ever increasing size of my girth which I've never totally lost. I can hardly be described as svelte — in fact I'm more than twice the weight I was when I was admitted to Sefton General in 1968. Mind you, I was only 14. My golf, incidentally, remains absolutely average because I don't play often enough.

Every year, Childwall Golf Club holds its golfing stag weekend at various golf clubs throughout the country. Most of the participants are damned good golfers, while I have more wooden spoons than Mary Berry. Despite this, socially it is an amazing, never-to-be-missed event. Even if I am not in their league as a player, at the dinner table and at the bar I certainly keep up with them.

I started this book at the moment when my life changed forever. I'd like to end it at another significant moment. This was a moment when I was able to give thanks for the life I ended up living.

In 2017, Frank Joseph first mentioned that I would soon be eligible for the Alan Nabarro Medal, which is given to people who have lived 50 years with diabetes, and that he would like to recommend me for it. But I assumed he was joking and forgot all about it, but he phoned me up and said, "Look, the anniversary is on 16 January 2018. Would you be interested in it?

I said, "Of course, I'd be interested in it."

And so it was November 2018 by the time it came round. What a proud and emotional experience my award ceremony was! Professor Frank presented me with my impressive-looking medal, and this was followed by a fantastic afternoon tea laid on by Diabetes UK and Spire Hospital Liverpool, the former Lourdes Hospital.

The tea included cream cakes with jam, and copious amounts of sandwiches. I felt guilty wanting to eat such lovely sugar-filled food, but Professor Frank laughed and said, "Eat what you like! You're a Type 1 diabetic."

So I got my flexipen out and enjoyed every morsel of that memorable afternoon tea surrounded by my closest friends, including Richard Lewis and Max Steinberg, plus my beautiful family of Nichola, Ella, Francesca, and Natasha.

And, at the end of my speech, I said, "I look forward, Good Lord willing, to seeing you all here again, 10 years from today, when I receive my 60 years award." I meant it, too. The Lawrence Award follows the Nabarro Award at 60 years, and the 70-year award is named after the author HG Wells (RD Lawrence and HG Wells were the founders of the Diabetic Association, now known as Diabetes UK). I fully intend to receive both of them.

However, I took a moment out to thank my lucky stars once again that this was 2018, and not 100 years earlier, when I wouldn't have survived 50 weeks, let alone 50 years.

Thank God for those heroic pioneers, who spent decades researching insulin, including the dogs whose lives were sacrificed so that experiments could be carried out, resulting eventually in the discovery in 1921 that has saved millions of lives, including mine.

And thank God for Dr Heinz Fuld, who I last met at Lourdes Hospital, under the roof of which I received my Nabarro Award. Without his diagnosis and guidance, I would not be here today.

But a final word to all diabetics worldwide: our condition need not be life-threatening as long as you don't let it dominate your life. Your fate is mainly in your own hands, so do what I've done. Get busy living.

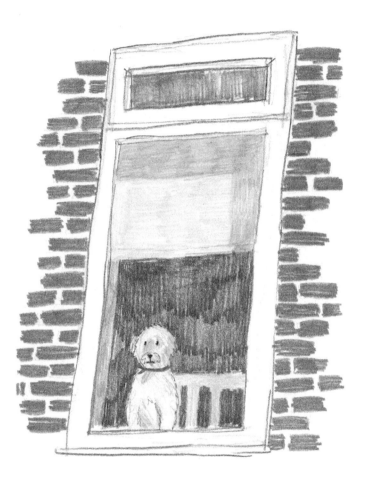

Index

Printed in Great Britain
by Amazon